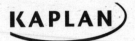

NCLEX® MEDICATION REVIEW

300+ MEDS YOU NEED TO KNOW FOR THE EXAM

TENTH EDITION

T0054428

Contributing writers: Margaret A. Tiemann, BS, RN; Barbara H. Arnoldussen, BS, RN, MBA; Jenny Collins, RN, MSN, MBA; Cheryl Martin, PhD, RNC-E, WHNP-E, CNE; Rebecca Potter, PhD, RN

Published by Kaplan North America, LLC dba Kaplan Publishing
1515 West Cypress Creek Road
Fort Lauderdale, Florida 33309

ISBN Retail: 978-1-5062-8993-9

ISBN Course: 978-1-5062-8994-6

Kaplan North America, LLC print books are available at special quantity discounts to use for sales promotions, employee premiums, or educational purposes. For more information or to purchase books, please call the Simon & Schuster special sales department at 866-506-1949.

TABLE OF CONTENTS

Ten Steps for Mastering the Medications on the NCLEX iv
Allergy and Asthma Medications. 1
Analgesics 9
Anesthetics 25
Anticoagulants. 25
Anticonvulsants. 33
Anti-Infectives 43
Anti-Inflammatory Medications 71
Antineoplastics 75
Antiplatelet Medications 79
Cardiovascular Medications. 83
Dermatologicals 129
Diabetic Medications 133
Gastrointestinal Medications. 145
Genitourinary Medications. 169
Herbal Supplements 177
Hormones/Synthetic Substitutes/Modifiers 187
Mental Health Medications. 191
Musculoskeletal Medications. 223
Neurological Medications. 235
Ophthalmics. 241
Otic Medications 249
Respiratory Medications 251
Treatment/Replacement. 261
Vaccinations 277
Vasoactive Medications. 289
Women's Health 297

Appendixes
Appendix A: Controlled Substance Schedules 305
Appendix B: Special Considerations 306
Appendix C: Common Medical Abbreviations. 307

Index
Index of Generic Medication Names 316

TEN STEPS FOR MASTERING
THE MEDICATIONS ON THE NCLEX

The best way to use this book to study for your nursing boards is to have a specific plan of attack! Then you can approach the sizable task of learning about medications with confidence.

1. Get your mind set for future success.

Focus on the fact that, after you pass the NCLEX and become a licensed registered nurse (*not* "if you pass"), you will be using the information you learned in this book in your daily life, both personal and work.

You will be using medication information every day. Likewise, you need to study these go-to medications every day, even if it's only in short bursts. Good news: This book is designed to be studied piecemeal. For example, if you want to review the whole book over 4 weeks, plan on a chapter a day. That lets you read the 26 chapters one medication category at a time.

Schedule time in your calendar for formal study every day. Don't rely on your previous experience of passing exams by pulling exhausting all-nighters. Do picture your study as gaining a solid understanding of concepts useful for your entire career.

2. Understand the book's flashcard format.

Think of the arrangement of information in this book as your two-sided master slide templates.

On the right-hand page, medications are arranged alphabetically under 26 medication categories. Each category tells which body system or medical condition the medication targets. Subcategories group medications with similar desired action within that body system or for that medical condition.

GENERIC NAME

(phonetic pronunciation guide)

Purpose: why the medication is given for a specific set of diseases or clinical conditions

Front flashcard information

For example, the first medication category, "Allergy and Asthma Medications," divides 9 medications under these headings:

- Antihistamines (5 meds listed alphabetically by generic name)
- Corticosteroids (4 meds listed alphabetically by generic name)

ADVERSE EFFECTS

First adverse effect
Second adverse effect, etc.

NURSING CONSIDERATIONS

- Information about medication pharmacodynamics (how the human body responds to a medication) and pharmacokinetics (how a medication behaves in the human body)
- Boxed warnings communicating serious safety risks
- Other nursing considerations
- Key client education highlights
- Rx or OTC (or both); controlled substance schedule (if applicable)

Back flashcard information

The nursing profession is about action. Therefore, the left-hand page focuses on the most critical nursing implications for you to learn. These can be summarized as "go" or "no-go" decisions for 2 situations:

- A specific adverse effect signals a medical condition that is severe enough to warrant calling the provider immediately.

- A vital sign such as pulse or respirations directs the nurse to withhold a medication (e.g., no digoxin if the client's pulse is under 60 bpm).

New in this edition, black box warnings (or boxed warnings) from the U.S. Food and Drug Administration (FDA) appear surrounded by a black border for easy visual identification. These warnings communicate rare but dangerous adverse effects and important instructions for safe use of the medication.

To build a firm mental connection between medication facts, talk to yourself! First, pronounce the generic name while looking at the phonetic pronunciation guide. Then, say the generic name again, while looking at the medication category and subcategory. Engaging 3 learning channels at once (looking, talking, and listening) promotes active learning and enhances your recall.

3. Keep your focus on the medication triangle.

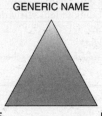

GENERIC NAME

PURPOSE   MEDICATION CATEGORY

Knowing the *purpose* for which the medication is designed allows you to accurately match client and medication. It firmly links the medication to the mental connections you established connecting the *generic name* with the *medication category*.

4. Consider both paper and people companionship.

This small book has purposely been sized to fit into a pocket or purse. Take it with you everywhere you go—think of it as your new, rectangular BFF.

Waiting in line can become an opportunity to review one medication category. Counting down the minutes until the microwave rings is enough time to look at another medication category.

If you know a fellow student who is as motivated as you are, talk to that person about setting up a "buddy system" where you can review your latest learning with each other. Make it a game: Quiz each other, *Jeopardy!* style, with one person giving the generic name and the other person guessing the purpose of that medication. You may be surprised by how these games energize you to prepare and remember.

5. Record your progress and thoughts.

By keeping track of your steps forward, you will enjoy 2 benefits: remembering where you left off, and marking the milestones of your journey. When you feel confident that you can recall the information up to a certain point in the book, mark it in some way that signals to you, "Done."

Make your messages to yourself obvious. What will communicate "Read here" or "Completed!" to you—a handwritten note? Folding over the corner of each completed page? Check marks in the margins? Remember: This is your book. Personalize it to work best for *you*.

Other additions that may help you focus on the material: circling or underlining key words, using a highlighter to enliven the facts you need with bright color, or mapping out similarities and differences of comparable medications in hand-drawn diagrams or tables. The more you interact with the material, the better you will be able to apply it.

6. Be alert for medication groupings.

The same suffix used in 2 or more medications hints at similarities in medication category and subcategory. Take the hint! As you go through the book, be alert for these "family" groupings, and chart them in your active study. Here is an example you can follow:

Suffix	Medication Category	Medication Subcategory	Generic Names
–afil	Genitourinary	Erectile dysfunction	Silden**afil** Tadal**afil** Varden**afil**
–asone	Allergy and asthma	Corticosteroids	Beclometh**asone** Flutic**asone** Momet**asone**
–azosin	Cardiovascular	Alpha blockers	Dox**azosin** Pr**azosin** Ter**azosin**
–cillin	Anti-infectives	Antibiotics: Penicillins	Amoxi**cillin** Ampi**cillin** Pipera**cillin**
–dipine	Cardiovascular	Calcium channel blockers	Amlo**dipine** Nife**dipine**
–olol	Cardiovascular	Beta blockers	Aten**olol** Metopr**olol** Propran**olol**

Suffix	Medication Category	Medication Subcategory	Generic Names
–pam	Mental health	Benzodiazepines	Clonaze**pam** Diaze**pam** Loraze**pam**
–pril	Cardiovascular	ACE inhibitors	Benaze**pril** Capto**pril** Enala**pril** Lisino**pril**
–romycin	Anti-infectives	Macrolides	Azith**romycin** Clarith**romycin** Eryth**romycin**
–statin	Cardiovascular	Antilipemic	Atorva**statin** Lova**statin** Prava**statin** Rosuva**statin** Simva**statin**
–tidine	Gastrointestinal	H_2 antagonists	Cime**tidine** Famo**tidine**
–vir	Anti-infectives	Antiviral	Acyclo**vir** Oseltami**vir** Valacyclo**vir**

7. Don't worry about brand names.

You will not see any trade/brand names on your NCLEX. The National Council of State Boards of Nursing, Inc., which develops the exam, strives for consistency over time—a stance that favors either the generic name or the medication category/subcategory. Trade and brand names are at the discretion of the many pharmaceutical manufacturing companies that produce them. *Trade and brand names can change.* Generic names are more stable, and thus are used by the National Council.

8. Do study herbal supplements.

Expect to see herbal supplements on your NCLEX. The National Council has added these to the detailed test plans for RN and PN testing. Herbal supplements may interfere with medications or cause difficulties when used in certain circumstances—and more people are using them. As a future nurse, you need to understand their implications for your clients. Some of the most widely used supplements are included in this book.

9. Take a quick final review.

Shortly before Test Day, pick up this book once again. Even if you only have the opportunity to look at the table of contents, doing so will refresh your memory before you take the NCLEX.

10. Get ready to celebrate!

Once you've passed the exam, keep this book as a souvenir of that fact that you earned your place in the ranks of registered nurses!

Additional resources available at
kaptest.com/nclex/free/nclex-practice

K

CETIRIZINE HCL
(se-<u>teer</u>-a-zeen)

Purpose: relief of seasonal allergic rhinitis symptoms

• •

DIPHENHYDRAMINE
(dye-fen-<u>hye</u>-dra-meen)

*Purpose: relief of allergy symptoms, rhinitis, and motion sickness;
treatment of insomnia*

ADVERSE EFFECTS

Drowsiness
Dry mouth

Headache
Constipation

NURSING CONSIDERATIONS

- Relief of perennial allergic rhinitis caused by molds, animal dander, other allergens
- Avoid alcohol during cetirizine therapy
- Call provider immediately for difficulty breathing or swallowing
- Notify provider for hydroxyzine allergy
- OTC

• •

ADVERSE EFFECTS

Dizziness, drowsiness
Palpitations, hypotension
Blurred vision
Nausea, diarrhea
Dysuria

Urinary retention
Thrombocytopenia
Photosensitivity
Chest tightness, wheezing

NURSING CONSIDERATIONS

- PO: peak 2–4 hr
- IM: onset 30 min, peak 2–4 hr
- Take with meals for GI symptoms; absorption rate may slightly decrease
- Take at bedtime only if using as sleep aid
- Should be discontinued 4 days before skin allergy tests
- Avoid driving and other hazardous activities if drowsiness occurs
- Avoid use of alcohol, CNS depressants
- OTC, Rx

FEXOFENADINE
(fex-oh-<u>fen</u>-a-deen)

Purpose: management of rhinitis and allergy symptoms

• •

HYDROXYZINE
(hye-<u>drox</u>-i-zeen)

Purpose: treatment of pruritus, preoperative anxiety, and postoperative nausea/vomiting; potentiation of opioid analgesics and sedation

ADVERSE EFFECTS

Drowsiness	Diarrhea	Itching
Headache	Vomiting	Hoarseness
Dizziness	Rash	Urinary retention

NURSING CONSIDERATIONS

- Avoid alcohol, CNS depressants
- Notify provider if taking erythromycin or ketoconazole
- If taking aluminum magnesium antacid, take antacid dose a few hours before or after this medication
- OTC, Rx

• •

ADVERSE EFFECTS

Drowsiness	Headache
Oropharyngeal dryness	Chest congestion
Dizziness	

NURSING CONSIDERATIONS

- PO: onset 15–30 min, duration 4–6 hr
- Avoid use with alcohol, CNS depressants
- Notify provider of diagnosis of glaucoma, ulcers, enlarged prostate gland, liver disease, hypertension, seizures, or hyperthyroidism
- Rx

K

LORATADINE
(lor-<u>at</u>-a-deen)

Purpose: management of seasonal rhinitis

• •

BECLOMETHASONE
(be-kloe-<u>meth</u>-a-sone)

Purpose: treatment of chronic asthma and of seasonal and perennial rhinitis; prevention of recurrence of nasal polyps after surgical removal

ADVERSE EFFECTS

Headache
Dry mouth
Diarrhea

Rash
Stomach pain
Tachycardia

NURSING CONSIDERATIONS

- Onset 1–3 hr, peak 8–12 hr, duration at least 24 hr
- Avoid alcohol, CNS depressants
- Take on empty stomach 1 hr ac or 2 hr pc
- OTC, Rx

• •

ADVERSE EFFECTS

Hoarseness
Oropharyngeal fungal
 infections
Headache
Sore throat

Dyspepsia
Rhinitis
Cough
Angioedema

NURSING CONSIDERATIONS

- Nasal spray: onset 5–7 days (up to 3 weeks in some clients), peak up to 3 weeks
- Inhaler: onset 10 min
- Use regular peak flow monitoring to determine respiratory status
- Rinse mouth after each use to prevent oral fungal infections
- Rx

K

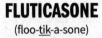

FLUTICASONE
(floo-<u>tik</u>-a-sone)

Purpose: treatment of chronic asthma and of seasonal and perennial rhinitis

· ·

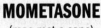

MOMETASONE
(moe-<u>met</u>-a-sone)

Purpose: treatment of chronic asthma and of seasonal or perennial rhinitis

ADVERSE EFFECTS

Hoarseness
Oropharyngeal fungal
  infections
Dyspnea
Headache

Nasal congestion, cold
  symptoms
Nausea, vomiting, diarrhea
Epistaxis, nasal irritation

NURSING CONSIDERATIONS

- Nasal spray: onset within 2 days, peak 1–2 weeks
- Use regular peak flow monitoring to determine respiratory
  status
- Rx

• •

ADVERSE EFFECTS

Hoarseness
Oropharyngeal fungal
  infections
Headache

Sore throat
Nasal congestion, cold symptoms
Nausea, vomiting, diarrhea
Muscle or joint pain

NURSING CONSIDERATIONS

- Nasal spray: onset few days, peak up to 3 weeks
- Use regular peak flow monitoring to determine respiratory
  status
- Rx

TRIAMCINOLONE
(try-am-<u>sin</u>-oh-lone)

Purpose: treatment of chronic asthma and of seasonal or perennial rhinitis

• •

ACETAMINOPHEN
(a-seet-a-<u>min</u>-a-fen)

Purpose: treatment of mild pain or fever

ADVERSE EFFECTS

Agitation
Oropharyngeal fungal
  infections
Headache

Blurred vision
Nausea, vomiting, diarrhea
Increased cough
Bronchitis

NURSING CONSIDERATIONS

- Nasal spray: onset few days, peak 3–4 days
- PO/IM: peak 1–2 hr
- Topical: apply to area several times per day
- Use regular peak flow monitoring to determine respiratory status
- Rx

ADVERSE EFFECTS

Anemia (long-term use)
Liver and kidney failure
Dyspnea (prolonged high
  doses)

Angioedema
Hives, itching

NURSING CONSIDERATIONS

- PO: onset less than 1 hr, peak 30 min to 2 hr, duration 4–6 hr
- Rectal: onset slow, peak 1–2 hr, duration 3–4 hr
- Signs of chronic poisoning: rapid, weak pulse; dyspnea; cold, clammy extremities
- Signs of chronic overdose: bleeding, bruising, malaise, fever, sore throat, anorexia, jaundice
- Take crushed or whole with full glass of water
- Take with food or milk to decrease GI upset
- Do not exceed maximum daily dosage
- OTC

ASPIRIN
(<u>as</u>-pir-in)

Purpose: management of mild to moderate pain or fever and TIA; antiplatelet prophylaxis of MI, ischemic stroke, and angina

• •

CELECOXIB
(sel-eh-<u>cox</u>-ib)

Purpose: management of acute chronic arthritis pain, relief of primary dysmenorrhea pain within 60 min

ADVERSE EFFECTS

Nausea, vomiting
Rash
Dyspnea

Tinnitus
GI bleeding

NURSING CONSIDERATIONS

- PO: onset 15–30 min, peak 1–2 hr, duration 4–6 hr
- Rectal: onset slow, 20–60% absorbed if retained 2–4 hr
- With long-term use, check for liver damage: dark urine, clay-colored stools, yellowing of skin and sclera, itching, abdominal pain, fever, diarrhea
- For arthritis, give 30 min before exercise; may take 2 weeks before full effect is felt
- Discard tablets if vinegarlike smell
- Do not give to children or teens with flulike symptoms or chickenpox; Reye syndrome may develop
- OTC

• •

ADVERSE EFFECTS

Fatigue
Anxiety, depression,
    nervousness
Nausea, vomiting, anorexia,
    dry mouth, constipation
Dyspnea

Back pain
Tachycardia
Dysuria
Palpitations
Bleeding

NURSING CONSIDERATIONS

- Onset 24–48 hr, duration 12–24 hr
- Can take without regard to meals
- Do not take if allergic to sulfonamides, aspirin, or NSAIDs
- Monitor for increased risk of MI and stroke
- Rx

IBUPROFEN

(eye-byoo-<u>proe</u>-fen)

Purpose: treatment of mild to moderate pain, reduction of inflammation

• •

MELOXICAM

(muh-<u>lox</u>-uh-kam)

Purpose: treatment of pain or inflammation caused by arthritis

ADVERSE EFFECTS

Headache	Dizziness	GI bleeding
Tinnitus	Blood dyscrasias	
Nausea, anorexia	Constipation	

NURSING CONSIDERATIONS

- Onset 30 min, peak 1–2 hr
- Used in rheumatoid arthritis, osteoarthritis, primary dysmenorrhea, gout, dental pain, musculoskeletal disorders, fever
- Take with food or milk to decrease GI symptoms
- Contact provider ringing/roaring in ears (possible toxicity)
- Contact provider if changes in urinary pattern, increased weight, edema, increased joint pain, fever, or blood in urine (may indicate kidney damage)
- Use sunscreen to prevent photosensitivity
- Avoid use with anticoagulants, aspirin, NSAIDs, alcohol (may precipitate GI bleeding)
- Monitor for increased risk of MI or stroke
- OTC, Rx

• •

ADVERSE EFFECTS

Dizziness	URI
GI upset	Flulike symptoms
Nausea, vomiting	GI bleeding

NURSING CONSIDERATIONS

- Take without regard to meals
- Monitor for increased risk of MI or stroke
- Rx

NAPROXEN
(na-<u>prox</u>-en)

Purpose: treatment of mild to moderate pain, reduction of inflammation

• •

BUPRENORPHINE/NALOXONE
(byoo-pra-<u>nor</u>-feen/na-<u>lox</u>-own)

Purpose: management of severe pain, treatment of opioid dependence

ADVERSE EFFECTS

GI bleeding	Vision changes	Tachycardia
Blood dyscrasias	Rash	GI disturbance
Tinnitus	Angioedema	
Insomnia	Jaundice	

NURSING CONSIDERATIONS

- Used in rheumatoid, juvenile, and gouty arthritis; osteoarthritis; primary dysmenorrhea
- Clients with asthma, aspirin hypersensitivity, or nasal polyps have increased risk of hypersensitivity
- May increase risk of MI or stroke
- Contact provider if black stools, flulike symptoms; blurred vision or ringing/roaring in ears (may indicate toxicity); changes in urinary pattern, increased weight, edema, increased joint pain, fever, or blood in urine (may indicate kidney damage)
- Avoid use with aspirin, steroids, alcohol
- OTC, Rx

• •

ADVERSE EFFECTS

Drowsiness	Headache
Sleepiness	Mental changes
Itching, rash	Hepatotoxicity
Blurred vision	Respiratory depression
Palpitations, tachycardia	Dependency

NURSING CONSIDERATIONS

- IM: onset 15 min, peak 1 hr
- IV: onset 1 min, peak 5 min
- SL: onset and peak unknown
- Avoid hazardous activities until reaction known
- Avoid alcohol and CNS depressants
- Sublingual route of administration may cause dental problems
- Rx C-V (parenteral), C-III (tablet)

CODEINE
(<u>koe</u>-deen)

Purpose: treatment of moderate to severe pain and of nonproductive cough

• •

FENTANYL
(<u>fen</u>-ta-nil)

Purpose: relief of moderate to severe pain

ADVERSE EFFECTS

Drowsiness, sedation

Nausea, vomiting, anorexia

Respiratory depression

Constipation

Orthostatic hypotension

Dysuria

Dyspnea

Seizures

Bradycardia

NURSING CONSIDERATIONS

- PO: onset 30–45 min, peak 1–2 hr, duration 4–6 hr
- IM/subQ: onset 10–30 min, peak 30–60 min, duration 4–6 hr
- Do not give if respirations are less than 12 per min
- Withdrawal symptoms may occur: nausea, vomiting, cramps, fever, faintness, anorexia
- Physical dependency may result from long-term use
- Avoid use with alcohol, CNS depressants
- Rx C-II, III, IV, V (depends on route)

• •

ADVERSE EFFECTS

Respiratory and circulatory depression

Coma, seizures, sedation

Dysphoria/euphoria, depression

Agitation, faintness, weakness

Visual disturbances, dizziness

Biliary colic, GI disturbance

Urinary retention/frequency

NURSING CONSIDERATIONS

- Black box warning: coprescribed with benzodiazepines or CNS depressants only if alternate treatments are unavailable
- Do not use with MAOIs, acute or severe bronchial asthma, or respiratory depression
- Tolerance and dependency may result from long-term use
- Available as transdermal patch
- Increased risk of serotonin syndrome
- Use with caution in pregnancy, breastfeeding, head injury, increased ICP or IOP, liver or kidney dysfunction, mental illness, emotional disturbance, drug-seeking behavior
- Rx C-II

K

HYDROCODONE/ACETAMINOPHEN
(hye-droe-<u>koe</u>-doan/a-seet-a-<u>min</u>-a-fen)

Purpose: treatment of moderate to severe pain

• •

HYDROMORPHONE
(hye-droe-<u>mor</u>-fone)

Purpose: treatment of moderate to severe pain and of nonproductive cough

ADVERSE EFFECTS

Dizziness
Drowsiness, sedation
Constipation
Nausea
Vomiting
Respiratory depression

Impairment of mental and
  physical performance
Rash
Pruritus
Palpitations

NURSING CONSIDERATIONS

- Use with CNS depressants and/or alcohol may result in addictive CNS depression
- Use with caution in clients with pulmonary considerations
- May be habit-forming
- Avoid alcohol during treatment
- Rx C-III

• •

ADVERSE EFFECTS

Drowsiness, sedation
GI disturbance, anorexia
Respiratory depression

Orthostatic hypotension
Confusion, headache
Rash

NURSING CONSIDERATIONS

- PO: onset 15–30 min, peak 30–60 min, duration 4–6 hr
- IM: onset 15 min, peak 30–60 min, duration 4–5 hr
- IV: onset 10–15 min, peak 15–30 min, duration 2–3 hr
- SubQ: onset 15 min, peak 30–90 min, duration 4 hr
- Rectal: duration 6–8 hr
- Do not give if respirations are less than 12 per min
- Older adult clients may require lower doses
- Avoid use with alcohol, CNS depressants
- Withdrawal symptoms may occur: nausea, vomiting, cramps, fever, faintness, anorexia
- Physical dependency may result from long-term use
- Rx C-II

K

METHADONE
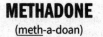
(<u>meth</u>-a-doan)

*Purpose: treatment of severe pain, detoxification, management of
narcotic addiction*

• •

MORPHINE

(<u>mor</u>-feen)

Purpose: treatment of severe pain

ADVERSE EFFECTS

Drowsiness, sedation

Confusion, headache

Respiratory depression

Rash

Constipation, cramps

Dysrhythmias

Orthostatic hypotension

Agitation

NURSING CONSIDERATIONS

- PO: onset 30–60 min, peak 30–60 min, duration 4–6 hr; with continuous dosing, duration of action may increase to 22–48 hr
- Do not give if respirations are less than 12 per min
- Avoid use with alcohol, CNS depressants
- Withdrawal symptoms may occur: nausea, vomiting, cramps, fever, faintness, anorexia
- Physical dependency may result from long-term use
- Rx C-II

• •

ADVERSE EFFECTS

Respiratory
depression

Euphoria

Bradycardia

Orthostatic
hypotension

Diaphoresis

Sedation

Urticaria

NURSING CONSIDERATIONS

- Continuous dosing more effective than prn; mazy be given by PCA
- PO: onset 15–60 min, peak 30–60 min, duration 3–6 hr
- IM: onset 10–15 min, peak 30–50 min, duration 2–4 hr (usually 3)
- IV: onset less than 5 min, peak 18 min, duration 3–6 hr
- SubQ: onset 10–15 min, peak 30–50 min, duration 2–4 hr (usually 3)
- Physical dependency may result from long-term use; possible withdrawal symptoms: vomiting, cramps, fever, faintness, anorexia
- Monitor for increased respiratory and CNS depression when given with cimetidine, clomipramine, nortriptyline, or amitriptyline
- Rx C-II

OXYCODONE
(ox-i-<u>koe</u>-doan)

Purpose: treatment of moderate to severe pain

TRAMADOL
(<u>tram</u>-a-dole)

Purpose: management of moderate to severe pain and chronic pain

ADVERSE EFFECTS

Drowsiness, sedation
Nausea, vomiting, anorexia
Respiratory depression
Constipation
Confusion, headache

Rash
Euphoria
Urinary retention
Orthostatic hypotension
Palpitations

NURSING CONSIDERATIONS

- PO: peak 30–60 min, duration 4–6 hr
- Controlled-release: peak 2–3 hr, duration 12 hr
- Do not give if respirations are less than 12 per min
- Avoid use with alcohol, CNS depressants
- Withdrawal symptoms may occur: nausea, vomiting, cramps, fever, faintness, anorexia
- Physical dependency may result from long-term use
- Rx C-II (controlled-release)

• •

ADVERSE EFFECTS

Dizziness, confusion
Headache
Orthostatic hypotension
Abnormal ECG
Visual disturbances

Nausea, vomiting
GI bleeding
Urinary retention/frequency
Rash
Respiratory depression

NURSING CONSIDERATIONS

- Give with antiemetic for nausea, vomiting
- Do not give with benzodiazepine or CNS depressant
- May cause serotonin syndrome, neuroleptic malignant syndrome
- Take with or without food
- Avoid OTC meds unless approved by provider
- Physical dependency may result from long-term use
- Rx C-IV

PROPOFOL
(<u>pro</u>-puh-fole)

*Purpose: general anesthesia and monitored anesthesia care (MAC),
sedation of intubated ICU clients*

• •

APIXABAN
(a-<u>pix</u>-a-ban)

*Purpose: prevention of clots; treatment of pulmonary embolism, deep
vein thrombosis, DIC, unstable angina, MI, atrial fibrillation, heparin-
induced thrombocytopenia, and heparin-induced thrombosis*

ADVERSE EFFECTS

Dystonic or choreiform movements

Bradycardia

Hypotension, hypertension

Decreased cardiac output

Hyperlipidemia

Increased serum triglyceride levels

Apnea, respiratory acidosis

Rash, pruritus

Burning or stinging at injection site

NURSING CONSIDERATIONS

- Administer into larger veins
- Do not infuse through a filter
- Allow 3–5 min between dosage adjustments
- Incompatible with other IV meds, blood, plasma
- Use with caution with soy or egg allergy
- Prolonged use may turn urine green
- Assess CNS function daily, discontinue gradually
- Teach to use caution when performing activities after use
- Abnormal dreams or anesthesia awareness may occur
- Rx

• •

ADVERSE EFFECTS

Bleeding

Hypersensitivity reactions

Thrombocytopenia

Increased liver enzymes

NURSING CONSIDERATIONS

- Do not give to clients with bleeding potential
- Contraindicated in aneurysm, active bleeding, hemorrhage, blood dyscrasias, hemophilia, hypertension, pericardial effusions, pericarditis
- Older adult clients may require lower doses
- Use with caution in severe diabetes, kidney impairment, severe trauma, ulcerations, vasculitis, pregnancy
- Avoid in breastfeeding due to increased risk of bleeding in infants (vitamin K deficiency)
- Stop med before surgery
- Increased risk for thrombus after discontinuing med
- Rx

DABIGATRAN
(da-<u>big</u>-a-tran)

Purpose: prevention of stroke in clients with nonvalvular atrial fibrillation, deep vein thrombosis, and pulmonary embolism

• •

ENOXAPARIN
(ee-<u>noks</u>-a-par-in)

Purpose: prevention and treatment of deep vein thrombosis

ADVERSE EFFECTS

Dyspepsia
Abdominal discomfort
Epigastric pain

GI hemorrhage
Bleeding
Neurological impairment

NURSING CONSIDERATIONS

- PO: may take without regard to meals
- Do not crush or chew capsules
- Closely monitor for signs of bleeding
- Increased risk of bleeding when combined with aspirin, other antiplatelets, anticoagulants
- Stop med 24 hr before surgery
- Rx

• •

ADVERSE EFFECTS

Bleeding
Bruising
Injection-site hematoma

Injection-site ecchymosis
Increase in AST/ALT

NURSING CONSIDERATIONS

- SubQ; can be given IV during cardiac procedures
- Do not use in clients with a history of heparin-induced thrombocytopenia
- Use with caution in clients with impaired kidney function or morbid obesity
- Monitor client for neurological impairment
- Monitor closely for signs of bleeding or excessive bruising
- Stop med 12–24 hr before surgery
- Rx

HEPARIN
(<u>hep</u>-a-rin)

Purpose: prevention and treatment of deep vein thrombosis and pulmonary embolism

• •

Anticoagulants
Anticoagulants

RIVAROXABAN
(riv-a-<u>rox</u>-a-ban)

Purpose: treatment and prevention of deep vein thrombosis and pulmonary embolism, prevention of stroke in clients with nonvalvular atrial fibrillation

ADVERSE EFFECTS

Spontaneous bleeding
Tissue irritation/pain at
   injection site
Increased AST/ALT

Anemia
Thrombocytopenia
Fever
Rash

NURSING CONSIDERATIONS

- Therapeutic PTT at 1.5–2.5 times the control without signs of hemorrhage
- IV: peak 5 min, duration 2–6 hr (give over 1 min)
- Injection: give deep subQ, never IM (danger of hematoma); onset 20–60 min, duration 8–12 hr
- Antidote: protamine sulfate within 30 min
- Available as generic only
- Abrupt withdrawal may precipitate increased coagulability
- Assess for signs of hemorrhage
- Avoid aspirin-containing products, NSAIDs
- Wear medical information tag
- Rx

● ●

ADVERSE EFFECTS

Bleeding
Bruising
Pruritus
Syncope
Nausea

Hematoma
Elevated bilirubin
Elevated ALT/AST
Neurological impairment

NURSING CONSIDERATIONS

- Dose reduction required in kidney impairment
- PO: give doses greater than 15 mg with food; lower doses may be given without regard to food
- Stop med 24 hr before surgery
- Monitor closely for signs of bleeding or excessive bruising
- Monitor for epidural or spinal hematomas
- Rx

WARFARIN
(<u>war</u>-far-in)

Purpose: prevention and treatment of deep vein thrombosis and pulmonary embolism, treatment of atrial fibrillation

• •

ALTEPLASE
(<u>all</u>-tuh-plase)

Purpose: treatment of MI, stroke, pulmonary embolism, and peripheral vascular occlusion; patency restoration of thrombosed grafts and IV access devices

ADVERSE EFFECTS

Hemorrhage
Diarrhea
Rash
Fever

Angina syndrome
Anemia
Dermatitis
Jaundice

Elevated liver
enzymes
Anaphylactic
reactions

NURSING CONSIDERATIONS

- Therapeutic PT at 1.5–2.5 times the control, INR at 2–3
- Onset 12–24 hr, peak 1.5–3 days, duration 3–5 days
- Antidote: vitamin K
- Avoid foods high in vitamin K: many green leafy vegetables
- Do not interchange brands; potencies may not be equivalent
- Do not take any medication or herb without provider approval
- Avoid aspirin-containing products, NSAIDs
- Oral anticoagulants may cause red-orange discoloration of alkaline urine, interfering with some lab tests
- Wear medical information tag
- Rx

. . . .

ADVERSE EFFECTS

Bleeding
Dysrhythmia
Allergic responses

Nausea, vomiting
Fever
Ecchymosis

Hypotension
Bleeding at
puncture site

NURSING CONSIDERATIONS

- Give by IV infusion
- Use with caution after surgery or trauma
- Numerous interactions with other meds
- Monitor vital signs carefully
- Observe for bleeding
- Do not use in pregnancy (except in life-threatening situations)
- Use with caution in breastfeeding
- Rx

CARBAMAZEPINE
(kar-ba-<u>maz</u>-e-peen)

Purpose: management of seizures, trigeminal neuralgia, neuropathic pain, bipolar mania, and migraines

• •

DIVALPROEX SODIUM, VALPROATE, VALPROIC ACID
(dye-<u>val</u>-proe-ex, val-<u>proe</u>-ate, val-<u>proe</u>-ic acid)

Purpose: management of seizures and bipolar disorder, prophylaxis of migraine headache

ADVERSE EFFECTS

Myelosuppression
Agranulocytosis
Aplastic anemia
Dizziness,
  drowsiness

Ataxia
Diplopia, rash
Photosensitivity
Depression
Nausea

Vomiting
Dyspepsia
Stevens-Johnson
  syndrome
Suicidal thoughts

NURSING CONSIDERATIONS

- Monitor blood levels, CBC regularly, esp. during first 2 months; periodic eye exams
- Avoid driving and other activities requiring alertness the first 3 days
- Take with food or milk to decrease GI upset
- Urine may turn pink to brown
- Avoid abrupt withdrawal; discontinue gradually
- Avoid use with alcohol, CNS depressants, grapefruit products
- Inform provider before taking any new med or herbal supplement
- Rx

• •

ADVERSE EFFECTS

Sedation, headache
Mental status and
  behavioral changes
GI disturbance
Hepatotoxicity

Teratogenicity
Pancreatitis
Thrombocytopenia
Multiorgan
  hypersensitivity

Rash, alopecia
BP changes
Visual disturbances
SIADH
Dyspnea

NURSING CONSIDERATIONS

- Delayed-release products: peak blood level 3–5 hr, duration 12–24 hr
- Extended-release products: onset 2–4 days, peak blood level 7–14 hr, duration 24 hr
- Monitor blood levels, platelets, bleeding time, liver function tests
- Monitor for suicidal thoughts or behavior
- Abrupt withdrawal may precipitate convulsions
- Take with or immediately pc to lessen GI upset; swallow whole
- Wear medical information tag
- Rx

GABAPENTIN
(ga-ba-pen-tin)

Purpose: management of seizures, postherpetic neuralgia, and primary restless leg syndrome

LAMOTRIGINE
(la-<u>moe</u>-tri-jeen)

Purpose: management of seizures and bipolar disorder

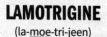

ADVERSE EFFECTS

Drowsiness
Ataxia
Diplopia

Rhinitis
Constipation
Memory problems

Back or joint pain
Edema
Diarrhea

NURSING CONSIDERATIONS

- Do not take within 2 hr of antacid use
- Avoid abrupt withdrawal after long-term use; discontinue gradually over a week to prevent convulsions
- Take without regard to meals; can open capsules and put in juice or applesauce
- Do not crush or chew capsules
- Use caution with hazardous activities
- Wear medical information tag
- Rx

• •

ADVERSE EFFECTS

Ataxia, dizziness
Headache
Diplopia, blurred
  vision
Rhinitis
Rashes

Loss of coordination
Nausea, vomiting,
  anorexia
Abdominal pain,
  dysmenorrhea
Mood changes

Irritability
Insomnia
Depression

NURSING CONSIDERATIONS

- Always notify provider of rashes; in pediatric clients, stop use at first sign of rash
- Take divided doses with meals or just after to decrease adverse effects
- Use caution with hazardous activities until stabilized
- Avoid abrupt withdrawal; stop gradually to prevent increase in frequency of seizures
- Wear medical information tag
- Rx

K

MAGNESIUM SULFATE
(mag-<u>nee</u>-zee-um <u>sull</u>-fate)

Purpose: prophylaxis of seizures with preeclampsia; treatment of eclampsia, acute nephritis in children, and hypomagnesemia

• •

PHENOBARBITAL
(fee-noe-<u>bar</u>-bi-tal)

Purpose: long-term management of seizures, management of febrile seizures, therapeutic sedation

ADVERSE EFFECTS

Muscle weakness
Flushing
Confusion, dizziness
Hypotension

Oliguria
Bradycardia
Decreased reflexes
Bradypnea
Hypophosphatemia

Hyperkalemia
Hypocalcemia
Hepatotoxicity

NURSING CONSIDERATIONS

- Given IM or IV
- Antidote: calcium gluconate
- Monitor blood pressure and reflexes
- Rx

ADVERSE EFFECTS

Drowsiness, lethargy
Rash
GI upset
Pupil constriction (initially)
Respiratory depression

Ataxia
Nightmares
Excitement in children
Hypotension, dizziness
Thrombocytopenia

NURSING CONSIDERATIONS

- IV: slow rate—resuscitation equipment should be available
- IM: inject deep into large muscle mass to prevent tissue sloughing (can give subQ), onset 10–30 min
- PO: onset 20–60 min, peak 8–12 hr, duration 6–10 hr
- Available as generic only
- Long-term use withdrawal symptoms: vomiting, sweating, abdomen/muscle cramps, tremors, possibly convulsions
- Vitamin D supplements are indicated for long-term use
- Use caution with hazardous activities until stabilized; drowsiness usually diminishes after initial weeks of therapy
- Rx C-IV

K

PHENYTOIN
(<u>fen</u>-i-toe-in)

Purpose: management of seizures

. . . .

PREGABALIN
(pre-<u>gab</u>-a-lin)

Purpose: treatment of neuropathic pain, postherpetic neuralgia, and fibromyalgia

ADVERSE EFFECTS

Drowsiness, ataxia
Nystagmus
Blurred vision
Rash
Hypotension

Lethargy
GI upset
Gingival
  hypertrophy
Depression

Urine discoloration
Thrombocytopenia
Hyperglycemia

NURSING CONSIDERATIONS

- PO: take divided doses, with or immediately pc, to decrease adverse effects
- IV administration may lead to cardiac arrest—have resuscitation equipment available; never mix in IV with any other med or dextrose
- Avoid abrupt withdrawal to prevent convulsions
- Do not use antacids or antidiarrheals within 2 hr of med
- Use caution with hazardous activities until stabilized
- Wear medical information tag
- Rx

• •

ADVERSE EFFECTS

Dizziness, tiredness,
  weakness
Headache
Nausea, vomiting,
  constipation
Flatulence, bloating

Mental status
  and behavioral
  changes
Lack of coordination
Increased appetite,
  weight gain

Back pain
Angioedema
Blurred vision
Tremor, twitching
Hypoglycemia

NURSING CONSIDERATIONS

- Take around the same time every day, 2–3 times daily; full therapeutic effects may require 4 weeks
- Do not crush or chew
- Avoid abrupt withdrawal after long-term use; discontinue gradually
- Avoid use with alcohol
- Use caution in potentially hazardous activities
- May increase the risk of suicidal thoughts or behavior
- Rx C-V

TOPIRAMATE
(toh-<u>pie</u>-ruh-mate)

Purpose: management of seizures, prophylaxis and treatment of migraines

• •

Anticonvulsants
Antimigraines

SUMATRIPTAN
(soo-ma-<u>trip</u>-tan)

Purpose: acute treatment of migraines

ADVERSE EFFECTS

Dizziness, drowsiness, fatigue

Impaired mental function

Speech problems

Nervousness

Nausea, anorexia, weight loss

Vision problems

Ataxia

Photosensitivity

Behavior problems, mood problems

NURSING CONSIDERATIONS

- Give without regard to meals
- Do not crush or chew
- Avoid abrupt withdrawal after long-term use; discontinue gradually to prevent seizures and status epilepticus
- Use caution with hazardous activities until stabilized
- Increase fluid intake to prevent formation of kidney calculi
- Notify provider immediately if experiencing periorbital pain or blurred vision
- Wear medical information tag
- Rx

• •

ADVERSE EFFECTS

Burning, tingling, numbness

Dizziness

Flushing

MI

Hypo/hypertension

Throat and nasal discomfort

Vision changes

Abdominal discomfort

Weakness, myalgia

Chest tightness, pressure

NURSING CONSIDERATIONS

- PO: take as soon as symptoms appear, swallow tablets whole
- Transdermal: apply to dry intact skin, discard after folding in half
- Onset 10 min to 2 hr, peak 10–20 min
- Ingestion of tyramine-containing foods (pickled products, beer, preservatives, chocolate) and caffeine may precipitate headaches
- Not to be used for more than 3–4 migraines per month
- Rx

AMIKACIN, GENTAMICIN, TOBRAMYCIN

(am-i-<u>kay</u>-sin, jen-ta-<u>mye</u>-sin, toe-bra-<u>mye</u>-sin)

Purpose: treatment of severe systemic infections of CNS, respiratory system, GI tract, urinary tract, bone, skin, and soft tissues

• •

AMOXICILLIN, AMPICILLIN, PENICILLIN

(a-mox-i-<u>sill</u>-in, am-pi-<u>sill</u>-in, pen-i-<u>sill</u>-in)

Purpose: treatment of respiratory, skin, gastrointestinal, and urinary infections and of otitis media and gonorrhea

ADVERSE EFFECTS

Use during pregnancy can result in bilateral congenital deafness

Ototoxicity
Nephrotoxicity
Neurotoxicity

Allergic reaction: fever, difficulty breathing, rash
Vertigo, tinnitus

NURSING CONSIDERATIONS

- IV over 30–60 min; IM by deep, slow injection; never subQ
- Carefully monitor blood levels: check peak 2 hr after med given; check trough at time of next dose
- Monitor for signs of superinfection (diarrhea, URI, coated tongue)
- Gentamicin available as generic only
- Encourage 8–10 glasses/day of fluids
- Immediately report hearing or balance problems
- May cause fetal harm if used during pregnancy
- Rx

• •

ADVERSE EFFECTS

Allergic reactions: fever, difficulty breathing, skin rash
Kidney, liver, hematologic abnormalities

Nausea, vomiting, diarrhea
Urticaria, rash
Bone marrow suppression

NURSING CONSIDERATIONS

- Take careful history of penicillin reaction; observe for 20 min post IM injection
- Check for hypersensitivity to other meds, esp. cephalosporins
- PO for penicillin and ampicillin: take 1 hr ac or 2 hr pc to reduce gastric acid destruction of the med; not true for amoxicillin
- Ampicillin and penicillin available as generic only
- Take equally divided doses around the clock
- Continue med for entire time prescribed, even if symptoms resolve
- Rx

AMOXICILLIN/CLAVULANATE
(a-mox-i-<u>sill</u>-in/<u>klav</u>-yoo-la-nate)

Purpose: treatment of lower respiratory infections, sinus and skin infections, otitis media, pneumonia, and impetigo

• •

PIPERACILLIN/TAZOBACTAM
(pye-<u>per</u>-uh-sill-in/taz-oh-<u>bak</u>-tum)

Purpose: treatment of moderate to severe infections, appendicitis, peritonitis, and hospital-acquired pneumonia

K 45

ADVERSE EFFECTS

Headache, agitation
Insomnia
Nausea, diarrhea, vomiting
Increased liver enzymes
Oliguria

Vaginitis
Bone marrow suppression
Hypo/hyperkalemia
Hypernatremia
Respiratory distress

NURSING CONSIDERATIONS

- Shake suspension before administering each dose
- Can be mixed with drinks
- Give with meal to increase absorption and reduce GI effects
- Give at equal intervals around the clock to maintain blood levels
- Discard unused suspension after 14 days
- Nephrotoxic with high doses
- Rx

• •

ADVERSE EFFECTS

Headache, dizziness, insomnia
Agitation, anxiety, seizures
Cardiac abnormalities, edema
Blood abnormalities
GI disturbance

Pseudomembranous colitis
Candidiasis
Interstitial nephritis
Pruritus, rash, fever
Anaphylaxis, hypersensitivity

NURSING CONSIDERATIONS

- IV: infuse over 30 min; monitor for phlebitis at infusion site
- Cross allergies to cephalosporins, beta-lactamase inhibitors
- Incompatible with other meds
- May decrease effectiveness of contraceptives and vaccines
- Monitor for kidney failure, bacterial/fungal superinfection, serious skin reactions
- Closely monitor fever and rash in cystic fibrosis
- Monitor sodium intake, electrolyte levels, hematologic and coagulation parameters
- Rx

AMPHOTERICIN B
(am-fuh-<u>tair</u>-i-sin)

Purpose: treatment of life-threatening invasive fungal infections

• •

FLUCONAZOLE
(floo-<u>kon</u>-uh-zol)

*Purpose: treatment of vaginal, esophageal, and systemic candidiasis
and of cryptococcal meningitis*

ADVERSE EFFECTS

Blood, kidney, heart, liver
   abnormalities
GI upset
Hypokalemia
Skin irritation and thrombosis
   if IV infiltrates
Rash

Fever, chills
Malaise
Hypotension
Headache
Nephrotoxicity
Ototoxicity

NURSING CONSIDERATIONS

- Given IV
- Available as generic only
- Do not mix with other meds
- Monitor vital signs; report fever or change in function, esp. nervous system
- Injection site requires meticulous care and observation
- Potential benefits must be balanced against serious adverse effects
- Rx

• •

ADVERSE EFFECTS

Nausea
Headache
Abdominal pain

Diarrhea
Hepatotoxicity

NURSING CONSIDERATIONS

- Prothrombin time is increased after warfarin usage
- Monitor glucose levels, esp. in clients with diabetes mellitus
- Take missed dose as soon as noticed, but do not double dose
- Rx

HYDROXYCHLOROQUINE
(hye-<u>drox</u>-ee-<u>klor</u>-uh-kween)

*Purpose: management of lupus erythematosus, rheumatoid arthritis,
and malaria*

· ·

QUININE SULFATE
(<u>kwye</u>-nine)

Purpose: treatment of malaria

ADVERSE EFFECTS

Eye disturbances
Nausea, vomiting
Anorexia
Photosensitivity
Dizziness

Headache
Hypotension
Skin changes
Ototoxicity

NURSING CONSIDERATIONS

- Peak 1–2 hr
- Give at the same time each day to maintain blood level
- Give with meals to decrease GI distress
- For malaria, prophylaxis should be started 2 weeks before exposure and continue for 4–6 weeks after leaving exposure area
- Rx

- -

ADVERSE EFFECTS

Eye disturbances
Nausea, vomiting
Anorexia
Tachycardia

Hypotension
Thrombocytopenia
Tinnitus

NURSING CONSIDERATIONS

- Peak 1–3 hr
- May increase digoxin levels
- Take at the same time each day to maintain blood level
- Do not crush
- Do not use to treat leg cramps
- OTC, Rx

METRONIDAZOLE
(meh-troe-<u>nye</u>-da-zole)

Purpose: treatment of a wide variety of infections including trichomoniasis, giardiasis, and bacterial vaginosis

• •

Anti-Infectives
Antituberculars

ISONIAZID
(eye-soe-<u>nye</u>-a-zid)

Purpose: treatment and prevention of tuberculosis

ADVERSE EFFECTS

Headache	Abdominal cramps	Depression
Dizziness	Metallic taste	Blurred vision
Nausea, vomiting, diarrhea	Darkened urine	Neurotoxicity

NURSING CONSIDERATIONS

- IV: immediate onset, PO: peak 1–2 hr
- Topical available for dermatological use
- Treatment of both partners is necessary in trichomoniasis
- Do not drink alcohol or preparations containing alcohol during and 48 hr after use; disulfiramlike reaction can occur
- May be carcinogenic
- Rx

. . . .

ADVERSE EFFECTS

Peripheral neuropathy
Liver damage
Nausea, vomiting

NURSING CONSIDERATIONS

- PO/IM: onset rapid, peak 1–2 hr, duration up to 24 hr
- Available only as generic or in combination with other med
- Contact provider if signs of hepatitis: yellow eyes and skin, nausea, vomiting, anorexia, dark urine, unusual tiredness, or weakness
- Contact provider if signs of peripheral neuropathy: numbness, tingling, or weakness
- Monitor liver tests
- Do not skip or double doses
- Rx

RIFAMPIN
(rye-<u>fam</u>-pin)

Purpose: treatment of acute tuberculosis and acute UTI

• •

ABACAVIR/LAMIVUDINE
(uh-<u>bak</u>-uh-veer/la-<u>miv</u>-yew-deen)

Purpose: treatment of HIV infection

ADVERSE EFFECTS

Headache, dizziness, fatigue
Shock
Hypersensitivity
Visual disturbances
Epigastric pain

Pancreatitis
Pseudomembranous colitis
Nausea, vomiting, diarrhea
Kidney failure

Thrombocytopenia, leukopenia
Liver failure
Allergy symptoms
Flulike reaction

NURSING CONSIDERATIONS

- Available as oral suspension, capsules, injection
- May cause red-orange discoloration of body fluids; may stain contact lenses
- Use with caution in liver impairment, diabetes mellitus
- Monitor liver function tests
- Monitor for overdose
- Do not use in late-term pregnancy or breastfeeding
- May interfere with oral contraception; use alternative birth control
- Avoid alcohol during therapy
- Rx

• •

ADVERSE EFFECTS

Hypersensitivity
Fever
Rash
Neutropenia

Thrombocytopenia
Liver toxicity
Lactic acidosis

NURSING CONSIDERATIONS

- Contraindicated in HLA-B*5701-positive clients
- May increase weight and metabolic parameters
- Monitor for pancreatitis and liver disease
- Rx

ACYCLOVIR
(ay-<u>sye</u>-kloe-veer)

Purpose: treatment of herpes and varicella

• •

EMTRICITABINE/TENOFOVIR
(em-tra-<u>sye</u>-tah-bean/tuh-<u>noe</u>-fo-veer)

Purpose: treatment of HIV infection

ADVERSE EFFECTS

Headache
Blood dyscrasias
Nausea, vomiting, diarrhea
Thrombocytopenia purpura

Nephrotoxicity
Tremors
Lethargy

NURSING CONSIDERATIONS

- IV: onset immediate, peak immediate
- PO: absorbed minimally, onset unknown, peak 90 min
- PO: take without regard to meals with a full glass of water
- Do not break, crush, or chew capsules
- If dose is missed, take as soon as remembered, up to 1 hr before next dose
- Contact provider if sore throat, fever, and fatigue; could be signs of superinfection
- Rx

• •

ADVERSE EFFECTS

Depression
Anxiety
Difficulty falling asleep or
  staying asleep
Unusual dreams
Pain

Burning or tingling in the
  hands or feet
Heartburn
Weight loss
Hypersensitivity

NURSING CONSIDERATIONS

- Should not be taken with St. John's wort
- Avoid if pregnant or breastfeeding
- Not approved for treatment of chronic HBV infections
- Take with meals
- Report adverse effects
- Rx

OSELTAMIVIR

(oss-el-<u>tam</u>-i-veer)

Purpose: prevention and treatment of influenza

• •

VALACYCLOVIR HCL

(val-a-<u>sye</u>-kloe-veer)

Purpose: treatment of herpes zoster (shingles), genital herpes, herpes labialis (cold sores), and varicella

ADVERSE EFFECTS

Nausea	Headache
Vomiting	Fatigue
Dizziness	Cough

NURSING CONSIDERATIONS

- Used to treat uncomplicated acute flu symptoms in clients that are symptomatic for 2 days or less
- Should not be used as a substitute for influenza vaccination
- May be taken without regard to meals
- Rx

• •

ADVERSE EFFECTS

Nausea, vomiting, diarrhea	Dizziness
Abdominal cramps	Dysmenorrhea
Headache	Thrombocytopenic purpura
Rash	Increased AST

NURSING CONSIDERATIONS

- Clients should drink plenty of fluids during treatment
- Avoid sexual contact when lesions are visible
- Rx

CEPHALEXIN, CEFAZOLIN
(sef-a-<u>lex</u>-in, se-<u>faz</u>-oh-lin)

Purpose: treatment of upper and lower respiratory tract, urinary tract, skin, bone, and otitis media infections

• •

CEFUROXIME
(sef-yoor-<u>ox</u>-eem)

Purpose: treatment of lower respiratory tract, urinary tract, skin, bone, joint, and gonococcal infections and of septicemia and meningitis

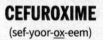

ADVERSE EFFECTS

Diarrhea
Anaphylaxis
Nausea
Rash
Headache

Nephrotoxicity
Dyspnea
Thrombocytopenia
Elevated liver function tests

NURSING CONSIDERATIONS

- Peak 1 hr, duration 6 hr (up to 12 hr with decreased kidney function)
- Possible cross allergy to penicillin
- May cause false positive of urine glucose
- Take for 10–14 days to prevent superinfection
- Rx

• •

ADVERSE EFFECTS

Nausea, vomiting, diarrhea
Headache
Rash

Elevated liver function tests
Nephrotoxicity
Thrombocytopenia

NURSING CONSIDERATIONS

- May cause increased BUN and serum creatinine
- May cause false positive urine glucose
- Possible cross allergy to penicillin
- Take for 10–14 days to prevent superinfection
- Rx

CEFDINIR, CEFTRIAXONE
(<u>sef</u>-di-neer, sef-try-<u>ax</u>-ohn)

Purpose: treatment of acute exacerbations of chronic bronchitis, sinusitis, pharyngitis, otitis media, tonsillitis, and skin infections

• •

CEFEPIME
(<u>sef</u>-e-peem)

Purpose: treatment of respiratory tract, urinary tract, skin, and bone infections

ADVERSE EFFECTS

Nausea, vomiting, diarrhea
Anorexia
Rash
Elevated liver function tests
Headache

Oral and vaginal candidiasis
Dizziness
Neurotoxicity
Thrombocytopenia

NURSING CONSIDERATIONS

- Available as generic only
- Do not give antacids or iron supplements within 2 hr
- May cause false positive for urine glucose
- Possible cross allergy to penicillin
- Take for 10–14 days to prevent superinfection
- Rx

• •

ADVERSE EFFECTS

Nausea, vomiting, diarrhea
Anorexia
Elevated liver function tests
Rash

Headache
Dyspnea
Nephrotoxicity

NURSING CONSIDERATIONS

- IV: peak 30 min
- IM: peak 2 hr
- May cause false positive for urine glucose
- Possible cross allergy to penicillin
- Rx

CIPROFLOXACIN
(sip-roe-<u>flocks</u>-a-sin)

Purpose: treatment of infections caused by E. coli and other bacteria and of chronic bacterial prostatitis, acute sinusitis, and postexposure inhalation anthrax

• •

LEVOFLOXACIN
(lee-va-<u>flocks</u>-a-sin)

Purpose: treatment of infections such as acute sinusitis, acute chronic bronchitis, pneumonia, and anthrax and of infections of the urinary tract, kidney, prostate, and skin

ADVERSE EFFECTS

Seizures

Headache, restlessness

Nausea, vomiting, diarrhea, abdominal distress, flatulence

Rash

Photosensitivity

Tendon rupture, muscle tear

Increased liver function test

NURSING CONSIDERATIONS

- Contraindicated in children less than 18 years of age
- Do not infuse with other meds
- Encourage 2–3 L/day of fluids
- May cause false positive in opiate screening tests
- Take 2 hr before or 6 hr after antacid or iron preparation
- Avoid caffeine
- Rx

• •

ADVERSE EFFECTS

Headache, dizziness

Nausea, vomiting, diarrhea

Stomach pain

Vaginal itching and/ or discharge

Tendon rupture or tendinitis

Insomnia

Hepatotoxicity

Photosensitivity, rash

Hallucinations, paranoia

Suicidal thoughts

Encephalopathy

Chest pain, palpitations

NURSING CONSIDERATIONS

- Infused injection over 60–90 min, once every 24 hr
- Available as generic only
- Monitor blood glucose; may cause hypoglycemia or hyperglycemia
- Monitor for peripheral neuropathy
- Rx

VANCOMYCIN
(van-ka-<u>my</u>-sin)

Purpose: treatment of Clostridioides difficile, *resistant staph infections, colitis, and staphylococcal enterocolitis; prophylaxis for endocarditis and dental procedures*

• •

CLINDAMYCIN
(<u>klin</u>-da-my-sin)

Purpose: treatment of infections caused by Staphylococcus, Streptococcus, *and other bacteria*

ADVERSE EFFECTS

Nephrotoxicity   Ototoxicity
Headache   Dyspnea

NURSING CONSIDERATIONS

- PO: poor absorption
- IV: peak 5 min, duration 12–24 hr
- IV: give over at least 60 min; do not infuse with other meds
- Give antihistamine if "red man syndrome": decreased blood pressure, flushing of face and neck
- Contact provider if signs of superinfection (sore throat, fever, fatigue)
- Check peak: 1 hr after infusion
- Check trough before next dose
- Encourage 2 L/day of fluids
- Rx

● ●

ADVERSE EFFECTS

Nausea, vomiting, diarrhea   Rash
Abdominal pain   Jaundice
Vaginitis

NURSING CONSIDERATIONS

- PO: peak 45 min, duration 6 hr
- IM: peak 3 hr, duration 8–12 hr
- May cause increase in AST, ALT, CPK
- Do not break, crush, or chew capsules
- Rx

AZITHROMYCIN
(a-zi-thro-<u>my</u>-sin)

Purpose: treatment of mild to moderate infections of the respiratory tract and skin and of nongonococcal urethritis, cervicitis, acute pharyngitis/tonsillitis, and community-acquired pneumonia

• •

CLARITHROMYCIN
(kla-<u>rith</u>-row-my-sin)

Purpose: treatment of respiratory, skin, and sinus infections

ADVERSE EFFECTS

Nausea, vomiting, diarrhea

Hearing loss

Dizziness, vertigo

Rash

Photosensitivity

Hepatotoxicity

Increased liver function tests

Vaginitis

Angioedema

Anemia

NURSING CONSIDERATIONS

- PO: rapid onset, peak 2.5–3.2 hr, duration 24 hr
- IV: rapid onset, peak end of infusion, duration 24 hr
- PO: don't take with antacids; can take with or without food
- Monitor for signs of superinfection (sore throat, fever, fatigue)
- If treated for nongonococcal urethritis or cervicitis, sexual partners also need treatment
- Increases effects of oral anticoagulants
- Rx

• •

ADVERSE EFFECTS

Nausea, vomiting, diarrhea

Headache

Taste abnormalities

Ventricular dysrhythmias

Vaginitis

Leukopenia

Rash

NURSING CONSIDERATIONS

- Available as generic only
- Treatment may be 7–14 days depending on organism and extent of infection
- Monitor for increase in theophylline, carbamazepine, and digoxin levels
- Monitor for signs of superinfection (sore throat, fever, fatigue)
- Take med with food
- Rx

ERYTHROMYCIN
(eh-rith-roe-<u>my</u>-sin)

Purpose: treatment of mild to moderate respiratory and skin infections, acne, conjunctivitis, chlamydia, and syphilis; newborn eye prophylaxis

• •

SULFAMETHOXAZOLE/TRIMETHOPRIM (CO-TRIMOXAZOLE)
(sul-fa-meth-<u>ox</u>-a-zole/try-<u>meth</u>-a-prim [koe-try-<u>mox</u>-a-zole])

Purpose: treatment of urinary tract infection, otitis media, chronic prostatitis, shigellosis, chancroid, and traveler's diarrhea

ADVERSE EFFECTS

Abdominal cramps
Pain at injection site
Nausea, vomiting, diarrhea
Rash

Anaphylaxis
Vaginitis
Dysrhythmias
Hepatotoxicity

NURSING CONSIDERATIONS

- IV: onset rapid, peak end of infusion, duration 6–12 hr
- PO: onset 1 hr, peak up to 4 hr, duration 6–12 hr
- PO: give 1 hr ac or 2 hr pc with full glass of water; avoid citrus juice
- Topical: apply small ribbon of ointment to inner eye
- Take at equal intervals around the clock
- Can be used in clients with compromised kidney function
- Monitor for signs of superinfection (sore throat, fever, fatigue)
- Rx

• •

ADVERSE EFFECTS

Hypersensitivity reaction
Blood dyscrasias
Photosensitivity
Nausea, vomiting, anorexia

Stomatitis, abdominal pain
Headache, fatigue
Bone marrow suppression
Increased BUN/creatinine

NURSING CONSIDERATIONS

- PO: with full glass water; if upset stomach occurs, take with food
- PO: take at equal intervals around the clock
- IV: infuse slowly over 60–90 min; flush lines at end of infusion to remove residue
- Monitor for hypersensitivity reaction; stop med at first sign of skin rash
- Never administer IM, rapidly IV, or by bolus injection
- Encourage 8–10 glasses/day of fluids
- Rx

DOXYCYCLINE HYCLATE
(dox-i-<u>sye</u>-kleen <u>hye</u>-klate)

Purpose: treatment of syphilis, gonorrhea, chlamydia, chronic periodontitis, acne, and anthrax; prophylaxis of malaria

• •

Anti-Inflammatory Medications
Corticosteroids

HYDROCORTISONE
(hye-dro-<u>kor</u>-ti-sone)

Purpose: treatment of severe inflammation, adrenal insufficiency, ulcerative colitis, collagen disorder, asthma, lupus, and COPD

ADVERSE EFFECTS

Photosensitivity

GI upset, diarrhea

Kidney, liver, hematologic abnormalities

Dental discoloration of deciduous (baby) teeth

Rash

NURSING CONSIDERATIONS

- Peak 1.5–4 hr
- Increases effects of anticoagulants
- Avoid during tooth and early development periods (4th month prenatal to 8 years of age)
- If GI symptoms occur, administer with food EXCEPT milk products or other foods high in calcium (interferes with absorption)
- Take with full glass of water; do NOT take within 1 hr of bedtime or reclining
- Rx

• •

ADVERSE EFFECTS

Depression

Flushing, sweating

Hypertension

Nausea, diarrhea

Hyperglycemia

Mood changes, euphoria

Blurred vision

Thrombocytopenia

NURSING CONSIDERATIONS

- Signs of infection masked by med, so check for elevated temperature, WBC count
- PO: take with food or milk
- IM: give deep into gluteal muscle, avoid deltoid, rotate sites, avoid subQ (may damage tissue)
- Rectal: for colitis, retain med for 60 min, onset 3–5 days
- Wear medical information tag
- Do not mix with other medicines
- Rx

METHYLPREDNISOLONE
(meth-ill-pred-<u>niss</u>-oh-lone)

Purpose: treatment of severe inflammation, shock, adrenal insufficiency, and collagen disorders; management of acute spinal cord injury and multiple sclerosis

• •

PREDNISOLONE
(pred-<u>niss</u>-oh-lone)

Purpose: treatment of severe inflammation, immunosuppression, neoplasms, and asthma

ADVERSE EFFECTS

GI hemorrhage	Poor wound healing	Thrombocytopenia
Hypertension	Hyperglycemia	Increased IOP
Circulatory problems	Mood changes	Nausea, diarrhea

NURSING CONSIDERATIONS

- PO: take with food or milk; peak 1–2 hr, duration 1.5 days
- IM: give deep into gluteal muscle, avoid deltoid, rotate sites; avoid subQ (may damage tissue)
- IM: peak 4–8 days, duration 1–4 weeks
- Monitor client weight, blood glucose, potassium
- Eat foods high in protein, calcium, vitamin D, potassium
- Contact provider if anorexia, difficulty breathing, weakness, dizziness (may occur during stress or trauma)
- Contact provider if black/tarry stools, slow wound healing, blurred vision, bruising/bleeding, weight gain, emotional changes
- Wear medical information tag
- Rx

• •

ADVERSE EFFECTS

Depression	Nausea, diarrhea	Tendon rupture
Hypertension, circulatory problems	Increased IOP	Poor wound healing
	GI hemorrhage	Hyperglycemia

NURSING CONSIDERATIONS

- PO: take with food/milk; peak 1–2 hr, duration 3–36 hr
- IM: give deep into gluteal muscle, avoid deltoid, rotate sites; avoid subQ (may damage tissue)
- IM: peak 1 hr, duration 4 weeks
- Monitor potassium, glucose, weight
- Eat food high in protein, calcium, vitamin D, potassium
- Contact provider if anorexia, difficulty breathing, weakness, dizziness (may occur during stress or trauma)
- Contact provider if black/tarry stools, slow wound healing, blurred vision, bruising/bleeding, weight gain, emotional changes
- Wear medical information tag
- Rx

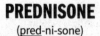

PREDNISONE
(<u>pred</u>-ni-sone)

Purpose: treatment of severe inflammation, immunosuppression, neoplasms, multiple sclerosis, collagen disorders, dermatological disorders, pulmonary fibrosis, and asthma

• •

CISPLATIN
(sis-<u>plat</u>-in)

Purpose: treatment of advanced bladder cancer, adjunct therapy in metastatic testicular and ovarian cancer

ADVERSE EFFECTS

GI hemorrhage
Hypertension,
  circulatory
  problems

Depression
Nausea, diarrhea
Abdominal
  distention

Hyperglycemia
Mood changes
Increased IOP

NURSING CONSIDERATIONS

- PO: take with food or milk, antacids
- PO: peak 1–2 hr, duration 24–36 hr
- Excessive consumption of licorice can increase risk of hypokalemia
- Eat food high in protein, calcium, vitamin D, potassium
- Contact provider if anorexia, difficulty breathing, weakness, dizziness; symptoms may appear during periods of stress or trauma
- Contact provider if black/tarry stools, slow wound healing, blurred vision, bruising/bleeding, weight gain, emotional changes
- Wear medical information tag
- Rx

• •

ADVERSE EFFECTS

Seizures
Peripheral
  neuropathy
Cardiac
  abnormalities
Ototoxicity
Blurred vision

Stomatitis
Nausea, vomiting
Kidney tubular
  damage
Thrombocytopenia,
  leukopenia
Sterility

Alopecia
Hypomagnesemia
Hypocalcemia
Hypokalemia
Hypophosphatemia
Fibrosis
Anaphylaxis

NURSING CONSIDERATIONS

- Available as generic only
- Use cytotoxic handling procedures
- Give antiemetic 30–60 min before treatment
- Monitor temperature every 4 hr
- Increase fluid intake to 2–3 L/day
- Rinse mouth 3–4 times/day for stomatitis
- Avoid vaccinations during therapy
- Rx

CYCLOPHOSPHAMIDE
(sye-kloe-<u>foss</u>-fuh-mide)

Purpose: treatment of cancer

• •

METHOTREXATE
(meth-oh-<u>trex</u>-ate)

Purpose: treatment of cancer, psoriasis, rheumatoid arthritis, and mycosis fungoides

ADVERSE EFFECTS

Headache, dizziness
Cardiotoxicity
SIADH
Stomatitis
Nausea, vomiting

Hepatotoxicity
Hemorrhagic crisis
Kidney tubular
  necrosis
Sterility

Leukopenia
Alopecia
Hyperuricemia
Pulmonary fibrosis

NURSING CONSIDERATIONS

- PO: take on an empty stomach
- Available as generic only
- Use cytotoxic handling procedures
- Avoid p.m. dosing
- Give antiemetic 30–60 min before treatment
- Monitor temperature every 4 hr
- Increase fluid intake to 2–3 L/day
- Rinse mouth 3–4 times/day for stomatitis
- Avoid aspirin, ibuprofen, vaccinations during therapy
- Rx

• •

ADVERSE EFFECTS

Nausea, vomiting,
  diarrhea
Anorexia
Alopecia, rash

Ulcerative stomatitis
Dizziness, headache
Kidney
  abnormalities

Hepatotoxicity
Thrombocytopenia
Lung disease
Infections

NURSING CONSIDERATIONS

- Available as generic only
- PO, IM, IV: onset 4–7 days, peak 7–14 days, duration 21 days
- Monitor for pulmonary toxicity, which may manifest early as a dry, nonproductive cough
- Avoid crowds and people with known infections
- Do not take with aspirin or other NSAIDs, which may cause GI bleeding
- Do not take with proton pump inhibitors
- Do not use during pregnancy
- Increase fluid intake to 10–12 glasses/day of fluids
- Rx

TAMOXIFEN
(ta-<u>mox</u>-i-fen)

Purpose: management of advanced breast cancer not responsive to other therapy in estrogen-receptor-positive clients

• •

CLOPIDOGREL
cloe-<u>pid</u>-uh-grel

Purpose: risk reduction for stroke, MI, peripheral arterial disease in high-risk clients, acute coronary syndrome, TIA, and angina

ADVERSE EFFECTS

Nausea, vomiting

Hot flashes, headache

Rash

Vaginal discharge

Irregular menses

Uterine cancer

Fluid retention

Depression, mood disturbances

Vision abnormalities

Chest pain

Stroke

Pulmonary embolus

NURSING CONSIDERATIONS

- Peak 4–7 hr
- Available as generic only
- To decrease GI upset, take after antacid, after evening meal, before bedtime, or take antiemetic 30–60 min ahead
- Vaginal bleeding, pruritus, hot flashes are reversible after stopping med
- Contact provider if decreased visual acuity, which may be irreversible
- Tumor flare (increase in tumor size and increased bone pain) may occur, but will decrease rapidly; may take analgesics for pain
- Rx

• •

ADVERSE EFFECTS

GI bleeding

Nausea, vomiting, diarrhea, GI discomfort

Depression

Bleeding, including life-threatening bleeding

Rash

Headache, dizziness

Edema

Chest pain

Glomerulonephritis

Liver failure

URI, bronchospasms

Arthralgia

NURSING CONSIDERATIONS

- Monitor blood studies in long-term therapy
- Report signs of unusual bruising, bleeding; it may take longer to stop bleeding
- Effectiveness dependent on individual metabolism
- Discontinue 5 days before elective surgery
- Take without regard to food
- Rx

PRASUGREL
(<u>prah</u>-soo-grel)

*Purpose: risk reduction for thrombotic events, prevention of cardiac
ischemic complications*

• •

TICAGRELOR
(tye-<u>ka</u>-grel-or)

*Purpose: risk reduction for thrombotic events and cardiac death after
MI, stroke, or stent placement*

ADVERSE EFFECTS

Serious bleeding

Thrombocytopenia

Anaphylaxis: rash, stomach
  pain, nausea, headache

Atrial fibrillation

Dyspnea, cough

Hypotension, hypertension

Hypercholesterolemia

Hyperlipidemia

Musculoskeletal pain

NURSING CONSIDERATIONS

- Contraindicated in pathological bleeding
- Not recommended for clients older than age 75
- Use with caution in clients weighing less than 60 kg
- Increased risk of bleeding after trauma, surgery, or liver impairment
- Discontinue 7 days before surgery
- Monitor for bleeding or bruising
- Take with aspirin
- Take without regard to food
- Do not break tablets
- Rx

• •

ADVERSE EFFECTS

Bleeding

Thrombocytopenia

Anaphylaxis: rash, stomach
  pain, nausea, headache

Atrial fibrillation

Dyspnea

Cough

Hypotension

NURSING CONSIDERATIONS

- Do not give if active bleeding or bleeding disorder, intracranial neoplasm, AV malformation, aneurysm, recent major surgery or trauma, severe uncontrolled hypertension, or thrombocytopenia
- Not recommended if stroke within past 2 years
- Avoid use in severe liver impairment
- Avoid use in pregnant or breastfeeding women: no research
- Discontinue 5 days before surgery
- May continue daily aspirin only if less than 100 mg/day
- Do not stop med abruptly
- Teach client about potential bruising/bleeding
- Rx

TICLOPIDINE HCL
(tye-<u>cloe</u>-pi-deen)

Purpose: prevention of stroke in high-risk clients

• •

BENAZEPRIL HCL
(ben-<u>ay</u>-ze-pril)

Purpose: treatment of hypertension

ADVERSE EFFECTS

Rash
Diarrhea
Bleeding
Decrease in WBCs
Thrombocytopenia

Nausea, GI distress
Purpuric rash
Headache, dizziness
Tinnitus
Hypercholesterolemia

NURSING CONSIDERATIONS

- Available as generic only
- Monitor blood studies in long-term therapy
- Monitor for signs of cholestasis (jaundice, dark urine, light-colored stools)
- Avoid all OTC products unless approved by provider
- Discontinue 10–14 days before surgery
- Take with meals or just after to decrease gastric symptoms
- Rx

• •

ADVERSE EFFECTS

Angioedema
Cough
Headache
Dizziness

Fatigue
Hyperkalemia
Nausea, vomiting, constipation

Hepatotoxicity
Increased kidney lab values

NURSING CONSIDERATIONS

- Often used in combination with thiazide diuretics
- Do not take in pregnancy; may cause fetal death
- Avoid salt substitutes containing potassium because of potassium-sparing effect
- Avoid nonprescription cough meds unless directed by provider
- Rx

K

CAPTOPRIL
(<u>kap</u>-toe-pril)

Purpose: treatment of hypertension, heart failure, left ventricular dysfunction after MI, and diabetic nephropathy

• •

ENALAPRIL
(e-<u>nal</u>-a-pril)

Purpose: treatment of hypertension, heart failure, and left ventricular dysfunction

ADVERSE EFFECTS

Bronchospasm,
  dyspnea, cough
Orthostatic
  hypotension

Dizziness
Loss of taste
Nephrotic syndrome

Bone marrow
  suppression
Hyperkalemia

NURSING CONSIDERATIONS

- Available as generic only
- Contact provider if fever, skin rash, sore throat, cough, mouth sores, swelling of hands/feet, fast or irregular heartbeat, or chest pain
- Take on empty stomach 1 hr ac or 2 hr pc; tablets may be crushed and mixed with juice or soft food for ease of swallowing
- Do not take in pregnancy; may cause fetal death
- Avoid changing positions (sitting/standing/lying) rapidly, esp. during the first few days before body adjusts to med
- Do not use OTC products (cough, cold, or allergy) unless directed by provider
- Avoid potassium supplements, potassium salt substitutes, potassium-sparing diuretics
- Rx

• •

ADVERSE EFFECTS

Headache
Dizziness,
  hypotension
Tachycardia,
  dysrhythmias

Tinnitus
Hyperkalemia
Angioedema
Persistent cough
Insomnia

Bone marrow
  suppression
Hepatotoxicity
Kidney failure

NURSING CONSIDERATIONS

- Contact provider if fever, skin rash, sore throat, cough, mouth sores, swelling of hands/feet, fast or irregular heartbeat, or chest pain
- Do not take in pregnancy; may cause fetal death
- Avoid changing positions (sitting/standing/lying) rapidly, esp. during the first few days before body adjusts to mediation
- Do not use OTC products (cough, cold, allergy) unless directed by provider
- Avoid potassium supplements, potassium salt substitutes, potassium-sparing diuretics
- May be crushed; give without regard to food
- Rx

86 K

LISINOPRIL
(lye-<u>sin</u>-oh-pril)

Purpose: treatment of mild to moderate hypertension, adjunctive therapy for systolic heart failure and acute MI

• •

DOXAZOSIN MESYLATE
(dox-<u>ay</u>-zoe-sin <u>mes</u>-i-late)

Purpose: treatment of hypertension and benign prostatic hyperplasia

ADVERSE EFFECTS

Headache, fatigue
Dizziness, vertigo
Nausea, vomiting, diarrhea

Hypotension
Tachycardia
Cough

Kidney insufficiency
Liver failure
Hyperkalemia

NURSING CONSIDERATIONS

- Do not take in pregnancy; may cause fetal death
- Avoid changing positions (lying/sitting/standing) rapidly
- May take without regard to food
- Avoid potassium supplements, potassium salt substitutes, potassium-sparing diuretics
- Rx

• •

ADVERSE EFFECTS

Dizziness, vertigo
Orthostatic hypotension
Headache
Tinnitus

Fatigue, malaise
Priapism (rare)
Nausea, vomiting, diarrhea

NURSING CONSIDERATIONS

- Can have first-dose syncope; maintain recumbent for 90 min
- Avoid changing positions (lying/sitting/standing) rapidly
- Use caution in potentially hazardous activities until stabilized
- Rx

PRAZOSIN HCL
(<u>pray</u>-zoh-sin)

Purpose: treatment of hypertension

• •

TERAZOSIN HCL
(ter-<u>ay</u>-zoh-sin)

Purpose: treatment of hypertension and benign prostatic hyperplasia

ADVERSE EFFECTS

Dizziness, drowsiness
Nausea, vomiting, diarrhea
Headache, vertigo
Palpitations

Syncope
Blurred vision
Nasal congestion

NURSING CONSIDERATIONS

- Onset 2 hr, peak 1–3 hr, duration 6–12 hr
- Can have first-dose syncope; take the first dose (and any increment) at bedtime, do not drive for 24 hr
- Full therapeutic effects may require 4–6 weeks of therapy
- Food may delay absorption
- Avoid changing positions (lying/sitting/standing) rapidly
- Check with provider before using OTC cold, cough, and allergy meds
- Rx

• •

ADVERSE EFFECTS

Dizziness, weakness
Headache, drowsiness
Nausea

Syncope
Blurred vision
Nasal congestion

NURSING CONSIDERATIONS

- Available as generic only
- Avoid changing positions (lying/sitting/standing) rapidly
- Can have first-dose syncope; take the first dose (and any increment) at bedtime, do not drive or operate machinery for 12 hr
- Check with provider before using OTC cold, cough, and allergy meds
- Rx

LOSARTAN
(loe-<u>sar</u>-tan)

Purpose: treatment of hypertension

. . . .

VALSARTAN
(val-<u>sar</u>-tan)

Purpose: treatment of hypertension and of HF in clients who cannot take ACE inhibitors; reduction of cardiovascular mortality post-MI in stable clients with left ventricular dysfunction/failure

ADVERSE EFFECTS

Dizziness, confusion	Diarrhea, anorexia	Photosensitivity
Insomnia	Dyspepsia	Alopecia, rash
Headache	Impotence	Hyperkalemia
Dysrhythmias, MI	Kidney failure	Hypoglycemia
Blurred vision	Thrombocytopenia	URI

NURSING CONSIDERATIONS

- Avoid hazardous activities until reaction is known
- Avoid grapefruit juice, alcohol, salt substitutes, OTC products
- Take without regard to meals
- Do not take in pregnancy; may cause fetal death
- Rx

• •

ADVERSE EFFECTS

Headache	Angioedema	Cough
Dizziness, vertigo	Abdominal pain	Hepatotoxicity
Hypotension	Nausea, vomiting,	Nephrotoxicity
Dysrhythmias	diarrhea	Hyperkalemia

NURSING CONSIDERATIONS

- Give on an empty stomach
- Determine if prescribed med is included in the voluntary recall list and follow guidance provided by the U.S. Food and Drug Administration (FDA)
- Do not take in pregnancy; may cause fetal death
- Take once daily for high blood pressure, twice daily for HF
- Avoid potassium supplements and salt substitutes containing potassium
- Rx

ISOSORBIDE DINITRATE
(eye-soe-<u>sor</u>-bide dye-<u>nye</u>-trate)

Purpose: treatment and prevention of chronic stable angina

• •

NITROGLYCERIN
(nye-troe-<u>gli</u>-ser-in)

Purpose: treatment of chronic stable angina; prophylaxis of angina pain, heart failure, and acute MI; controlled hypotension for surgical procedures

ADVERSE EFFECTS

Dizziness, orthostatic
  hypotension
Vascular headache, flushing

Drowsiness
Nausea, vomiting
Lightheadedness

NURSING CONSIDERATIONS

- PO: 1 hr ac or 2 hr pc for maximum absorption, but taking with food may reduce or eliminate headache
- Chewable tablet: chew well, hold in mouth for 2 min before swallowing
- SL: dissolve under tongue; do not eat, drink, talk, or smoke during use; go to ED if pain not relieved in 15 min
- Avoid changing positions (lying/sitting/standing) rapidly
- Use caution in potentially hazardous activities until stabilized
- Avoid alcohol, smoking, strenuous exercise in hot environment
- Wear medical information tag
- Rx

• •

ADVERSE EFFECTS

Postural hypotension
Nausea, vomiting

Headache, flushing, dizziness

NURSING CONSIDERATIONS

- Sustained-release: take every 6–12 hr on an empty stomach; onset 20–45 min, duration 3–8 hr
- SL: client sitting/lying should let tablet dissolve under tongue and not swallow saliva; onset 1–3 min, duration 30 min
- Spray: hold canister upright, spray on tongue (do not inhale), close mouth immediately; onset 2 min, duration 30–60 min
- IV: use infusion pump and special non-PVC tubing; onset 1–2 min, duration 3–5 min
- Ointment: spread on skin in thin uniform layer; onset 30–60 min, duration 2–12 hr
- Transdermal: apply to clean hairless area; rotate sites; onset 30–60 min, duration 12–24 hr
- Go to ED if pain not relieved with first tablet
- Wear medical information tag
- Rx

AMIODARONE HCL
(am-ee-<u>oh</u>-da-rone)

Purpose: management of ventricular dysrhythmias not controlled by first-line agents

• •

FLECAINIDE
(fleh-<u>kay</u>-nide)

Purpose: management of life-threatening ventricular dysrhythmias, sustained ventricular tachycardia, and atrial flutter/fibrillation

ADVERSE EFFECTS

Dizziness, fatigue, malaise

Anorexia, constipation

Nausea, vomiting

Bradycardia, hypotension

Corneal microdeposits

Photosensitivity

Hypo/ hyperthyroidism

Muscle weakness

Cardiac arrest

Peripheral neuropathy

Rash

Neurotoxicity

Pulmonary toxicity

Hepatotoxicity

NURSING CONSIDERATIONS

- IV requires continuous cardiac monitoring
- Assess for signs of pulmonary toxicity: rales/crackles, decreased breath sounds, pleuritic friction rub, fatigue, dyspnea, cough, pleuritic pain, fever
- Adverse effects may not appear for several days, weeks, or years and may persist for several months after stopping med
- Teach client to check radial pulse
- May increase ALT, AST
- Rx

• •

ADVERSE EFFECTS

Headache, dizziness

Blurred vision

Irritability, depression

Hypotension, bradycardia

Heart failure

Tachycardia

Tremors

Tinnitus

Nausea, vomiting, constipation

Change in taste

Impotence

Urinary retention

Leukopenia

Respiratory depression

NURSING CONSIDERATIONS

- Available as generic only
- May adjust dose every 4 days
- Reduce dosage as soon as dysrhythmia is controlled
- Take with meals to minimize GI upset
- Avoid changing positions (lying/sitting/standing) rapidly
- Do not skip or double doses; if dose missed, take as soon as possible within 6 hr of next dose
- Wear medical identification tag
- Rx

LIDOCAINE HCL
(<u>lye</u>-doe-kane)

Purpose: management of ventricular tachycardia and ventricular dysrhythmias during cardiac surgery

• •

PROCAINAMIDE
(proe-<u>kane</u>-a-mide)

Purpose: management of life-threatening ventricular dysrhythmias

ADVERSE EFFECTS

Hypotension, tremors
Blurred vision
Tinnitus
Respiratory depression/arrest
Confusion

Drowsiness, dizziness
Seizures
Bradycardia
Nausea, vomiting, anorexia
Rash, petechiae

NURSING CONSIDERATIONS

- Give oxygen; have resuscitation equipment available
- IV: use infusion pump; client on cardiac monitor
- Rx

- -

ADVERSE EFFECTS

Hypotension
Nausea, vomiting
Fever, rash
Dizziness

Bone marrow suppression
SLE syndrome
Confusion, restlessness
Angioedema

NURSING CONSIDERATIONS

- IV: use infusion pump; monitor BP every 5–15 min; on cardiac monitor; keep client recumbent
- IV: monitor CBC, blood levels, I&O, daily weight
- Available as generic only
- May increase alkaline phosphatase, bilirubin, AST, ALT
- Rx

QUINIDINE
(<u>kwin</u>-i-deen)

Purpose: management of atrial or ventricular dysrhythmias and of malaria

SOTALOL
(<u>soe</u>-ta-lole)

Purpose: management of life-threatening ventricular dysrhythmias

ADVERSE EFFECTS

Anemia
Hypotension, bradycardia
Nausea, vomiting, diarrhea
Headache, dizziness
Heart block

Tinnitus
Vision changes
Respiratory depression
Hepatotoxicity
Thrombocytopenia

NURSING CONSIDERATIONS

- May increase toxicity for digitalis
- Available as generic only
- Monitor ECG, BP, and pulse
- Increased risk of death if used for non-life-threatening dysrhythmias
- Avoid changing positions (lying/sitting/standing) rapidly
- Avoid use with alcohol, caffeine, smoking
- Wear medical information tag
- Rx

• •

ADVERSE EFFECTS

Fatigue, drowsiness
Weakness, dizziness
Visual changes
Bradycardia

Life-threatening
ventricular
dysrhythmias
Impotence

GI disturbance
Hyperglycemia
Dyspnea,
bronchospasms

NURSING CONSIDERATIONS

- PO: give 1 hr ac or 1 hr pc
- Administer first 3 days in hospital setting only
- Teach client to check radial pulse; if less than 50 bpm, hold med and contact provider
- Change positions (sitting/standing/lying) slowly
- Avoid activities that require alertness until med response known
- Contact provider if slow pulse, difficulty breathing, wheezing, rash, fever, sore throat, unusual bleeding or bruising
- Wear medical information tag
- Avoid alcohol, smoking, sodium
- Rx

CLONIDINE
(<u>kloe</u>-ni-deen)

Purpose: treatment of hypertension, severe pain in clients with cancer, and ADHD

• •

HYDRALAZINE HCL
(hye-<u>dral</u>-a-zeen)

Purpose: treatment of essential hypertension and hypertensive emergency

ADVERSE EFFECTS

Drowsiness, sedation

Severe rebound hypertension

Dry mouth and eyes

Hyperglycemia

Nausea, vomiting, constipation

Orthostatic hypotension

Impotence

Taste change

Dizziness

Headache

Rash

NURSING CONSIDERATIONS

- Apply patch to nonhairy area (upper outer arm, anterior chest), rotate sites, do not apply to scarred or irritated area
- Avoid changing positions (lying/sitting/standing) rapidly
- Avoid use with CNS depressants, OTC meds with stimulants
- Avoid high-sodium foods, alcohol, smoking, strenuous exercise in hot environment
- Wear medical information tag
- Rx

• •

ADVERSE EFFECTS

Headache

Palpitations, tachycardia, angina

Edema

Lupus erythematosus–like syndrome

Anorexia

Dizziness

Anxiety

Rash

Nausea, vomiting, diarrhea

Hepatotoxicity

Leukopenia

Orthostatic hypotension

NURSING CONSIDERATIONS

- Do not confuse with hydroxyzine
- Available as generic only
- Avoid changing positions (lying/sitting/standing) rapidly
- Contact provider if chest pain, severe fatigue, fever, muscle, or joint pain
- Rx

ATORVASTATIN CALCIUM
(a-<u>tor</u>-va-stat-in)

Purpose: reduction of cholesterol levels

● ●

EZETIMIBE
(e-<u>zet</u>-i-mibe)

Purpose: reduction of cholesterol levels

ADVERSE EFFECTS

Constipation
Abdominal pain
Nausea, diarrhea
Arthralgia

Impotence
Headache, insomnia
Increased liver enzymes
Lens opacities

NURSING CONSIDERATIONS

- Peak 1–2 hr
- Take without regard to food
- Avoid grapefruit products
- Contact provider immediately if unexplained muscle pain, tenderness, or weakness; in rare cases, med causes breakdown of skeletal muscle tissue, leading to kidney failure
- Rx

• •

ADVERSE EFFECTS

Diarrhea, abdominal pain
Joint pain, arthralgia

Fatigue, dizziness
URI, sinusitis

NURSING CONSIDERATIONS

- Peak 4–12 hr
- Ezetimibe is not a statin; can be used with a statin or alone; works by removing cholesterol from the small intestine (statins work in the liver)
- Contact provider immediately if unexplained muscle pain, tenderness, or weakness; in rare cases, med causes breakdown of skeletal muscle tissue, leading to kidney failure
- Take without regard to meals
- Rx

FENOFIBRATE
(fen-oh-<u>fye</u>-brate)

Purpose: reduction of cholesterol levels

• •

GEMFIBROZIL
(jem-<u>fye</u>-bruh-zill)

Purpose: reduction of cholesterol levels

ADVERSE EFFECTS

Fatigue, weakness
Insomnia
Depression
Hypo/hypertension
Nausea, vomiting,
  dyspepsia

Increased liver
  enzymes
Pancreatitis
Dysuria
Leukopenia
Photosensitivity

Rash
Weight gain
Myalgia
Cough

NURSING CONSIDERATIONS

- Contact provider if unexplained muscle pain, tenderness, or weakness; in rare cases, med causes breakdown of skeletal muscle tissue, leading to kidney failure
- Avoid changing positions (lying/sitting/standing) rapidly
- Rx

• •

ADVERSE EFFECTS

Fatigue, vertigo
Headache
Dyspepsia
Nausea, vomiting, diarrhea
Abdominal pain

Leukopenia
Rash, urticaria
Altered taste
Myopathy
Angioedema

NURSING CONSIDERATIONS

- Administer 30 min before a.m. and p.m. meals
- Monitor blood glucose, kidney/liver studies in long-term therapy
- Avoid alcohol, high-fat diet, smoking, sedentary lifestyle
- Rx

LOVASTATIN
(<u>loh</u>-vah-stat-in)

Purpose: reduction of cholesterol levels

• •

NIACIN (NICOTINIC ACID)
(<u>nye</u>-a-sin)

Purpose: treatment of pellagra, hyperlipidemia, and peripheral vascular disease

ADVERSE EFFECTS

GI disturbance:
pain, upset,
nausea, diarrhea
Flatus, constipation
Heartburn

Muscle cramps
Dizziness
Headache
Tremor
Blurred vision

Rash, pruritus
Photosensitivity
Increased liver
function tests

NURSING CONSIDERATIONS

- Onset 2 weeks, peak 4–6 weeks, duration 6 weeks
- Take with food; absorption is reduced by 30% on an empty stomach
- Contact provider if unexplained muscle pain, tenderness, or weakness; in rare cases, med causes breakdown of skeletal muscle tissue leading to kidney failure
- Avoid grapefruit products
- Rx

• •

ADVERSE EFFECTS

Headache
Nausea, vomiting
Postural hypotension
Myopathy
Flushing

Pruritus
Liver function test
abnormalities
Hyperglycemia

NURSING CONSIDERATIONS

- Flushing will occur several hr after med taken; will decrease over 2 weeks
- May be used in combination with simvastatin or lovastatin
- Take with meals to reduce GI upset; can add 325 mg aspirin 30 min before dose to reduce flushing
- Avoid changing positions (sitting/standing/lying) rapidly
- OTC, Rx

PRAVASTATIN
(<u>prav</u>-a-stat-in)

Purpose: reduction of cholesterol levels and risk of recurrent MI, treatment of atherosclerosis

• •

ROSUVASTATIN CALCIUM
(roe-<u>sue</u>-vuh-stat-in)

Purpose: reduction of cholesterol levels and progression of atherosclerosis, prophylaxis of cardiovascular disease and stroke

ADVERSE EFFECTS

Abdominal cramps, flatus
Heartburn
Constipation, diarrhea
Headache, dizziness, fatigue

Lens opacities
Kidney failure
Muscle cramps
Liver dysfunction

NURSING CONSIDERATIONS

- Peak 1–1.5 hr
- Take without regard to food
- Contact provider if unexplained muscle pain, tenderness, or weakness; in rare cases, med causes breakdown of skeletal muscle tissue leading to kidney failure
- Rx

• •

ADVERSE EFFECTS

Myalgia
Constipation, heartburn
Abdominal pain
Rash, pruritus
Nausea

Thrombocytopenia
Muscle cramps, arthralgia
Headache, dizziness
Kidney failure
Liver dysfunction

NURSING CONSIDERATIONS

- Client should keep tight control of diet during therapy
- Asian clients may require lower dose at initiation of therapy
- Contact provider if unexplained muscle pain, tenderness, or weakness; in rare cases, med causes breakdown of skeletal muscle tissue leading to kidney failure
- Take without regard to meals
- Rx

SIMVASTATIN
(<u>sim</u>-va-stat-in)

*Purpose: reduction of cholesterol, triglyceride, and lipoprotein levels;
  prophylaxis of MI and stroke*

• •

ATENOLOL
(a-<u>ten</u>-oh-lole)

*Purpose: treatment of mild to moderate hypertension and MI,
  prophylaxis of angina*

ADVERSE EFFECTS

Liver dysfunction
URI
Headache
Abdominal pain

Constipation
Nausea
Muscle cramps, myalgia
Hyperglycemia

NURSING CONSIDERATIONS

- May require lower dose at initiation of therapy
- Asian clients should not take niacin while taking simvastatin
- Take without regard to food
- Contact provider if unexplained muscle pain, tenderness, or weakness; in rare cases, med causes breakdown of skeletal muscle tissue leading to kidney failure
- Rx

• •

ADVERSE EFFECTS

Bradycardia
Postural
  hypotension
Bronchospasm in
  overdose

2nd- or 3rd-degree
  heart block
Cold extremities
Insomnia, fatigue
Dizziness

Mental changes
Nausea, diarrhea
Hypoglycemia
Impotence
Thrombocytopenia

NURSING CONSIDERATIONS

- Masks signs of hypoglycemia in clients with diabetes
- Check pulse; if less than 50 bpm, hold med and contact provider
- PO: take ac, at bedtime
- Do not stop abruptly; taper over 2 weeks
- Limit alcohol, smoking, sodium intake
- Rx

BISOPROLOL
(bis-<u>oh</u>-pro-lole)

Purpose: treatment of mild to moderate hypertension

• •

CARVEDILOL
(kar-<u>ved</u>-i-lole)

Purpose: treatment of hypertension, heart failure, LV dysfunction after MI, and cardiomyopathy

ADVERSE EFFECTS

GI upset
Dizziness, vertigo
Headache, fatigue
Bronchospasms, dyspnea

Postural hypotension
Impotence
Increased AST/ALT

NURSING CONSIDERATIONS

- Peak: 2–4 hr
- Therapeutic response in 1–2 weeks
- Available as generic only
- Teach client to check radial pulse
- Contact provider if signs of heart failure: difficulty breathing, night cough, swelling of extremities
- Do not stop med abruptly; may precipitate angina
- Do not use OTC meds with stimulants, such as nasal decongestants or cold meds, unless directed
- Avoid alcohol, smoking, sodium intake
- Rx

• •

ADVERSE EFFECTS

Dizziness, fatigue
Diarrhea
Postural hypotension
Impotence
Hyperglycemia
Heart failure worsening
Paresthesia

Bradycardia
Peripheral edema
Headache, insomnia
Increased liver enzymes
Thrombocytopenia
Bronchospasm

NURSING CONSIDERATIONS

- PO: take with food
- Tablet may be crushed or swallowed whole
- Do not stop abruptly; taper over 1–2 weeks
- Rx

METOPROLOL
(meh-<u>toe</u>-proe-lole)

Purpose: treatment of hypertension, acute MI, angina, heart failure, and cardiomyopathy

• •

PROPRANOLOL HCL
(proe-<u>pran</u>-oh-lole)

Purpose: treatment of stable angina, hypertension, supraventricular dysrhythmias, and acute MI; prophylaxis of migraine

ADVERSE EFFECTS

Bradycardia, palpitations
Nausea, vomiting, diarrhea
Hypotension, dizziness
Heart failure
Depression
Insomnia

Confusion, headache
Impotence
Bronchospasms
Rash, urticaria
Hypoglycemia

NURSING CONSIDERATIONS

- Check pulse; if less than 60 bpm, hold med and contact provider
- PO: may be taken with food, take at same time each day
- XL tablet must be swallowed whole
- Do not stop abruptly; taper over 2 weeks; may precipitate angina
- Do not use OTC products (nasal decongestants, cold preparations) unless directed by provider
- May worsen heart failure
- Rx

• •

ADVERSE EFFECTS

Weakness, fatigue
Hypotension, dizziness
Impotence
Bronchospasm
Bradycardia
Nausea, vomiting

Depression
Blurred vision
Hyper/hypoglycemia
Dysrhythmias
Thrombocytopenia
Arthralgia

NURSING CONSIDERATIONS

- Check pulse; if less than 50 bpm, hold med and contact provider
- PO: take with full glass of water at the same time each day
- Do not open, chew, or crush extended-release capsule
- Do not stop abruptly; taper over 2 weeks; may precipitate life-threatening dysrhythmias
- Do not use aluminum-containing antacid; may decrease absorption
- Rx

AMLODIPINE
(am-<u>loh</u>-di-peen)

Purpose: treatment of chronic stable angina, hypertension, and variant angina

. . . .

DILTIAZEM HCL
(dil-<u>tye</u>-a-zem)

Purpose: management of angina, vasospasms, hypertension, atrial fibrillation/flutter, and supraventricular tachycardia

ADVERSE EFFECTS

Flushing

Headache, fatigue

Nausea, vomiting

Abdominal pain

Somnolence

Peripheral edema

Nocturia

Sexual difficulties

Palpitations, bradycardia

Cough, dyspnea

NURSING CONSIDERATIONS

- May be taken without regard to meals
- Consult provider before taking nonprescription cough remedies
- Check pulse; if less than 50 bpm, hold med and contact provider
- Avoid changing positions (lying/sitting/standing) rapidly
- Avoid grapefruit juice
- Rx

• •

ADVERSE EFFECTS

Edema

Nausea, constipation

Rash

Photosensitivity

Headache, dizziness

Fatigue, drowsiness

Bradycardia, palpitations

Increased liver enzymes

Kidney failure

Nocturia

Heart failure, dysrhythmias

NURSING CONSIDERATIONS

- PO: take on an empty stomach with a full glass of water
- Monitor BP during dosage adjustments
- Teach client how to measure and document radial pulse; if less than 50 bpm, hold dose and notify provider
- Avoid hazardous activities until stabilized on med
- Do not crush, chew, or break
- Do not stop abruptly
- Avoid grapefruit juice
- Rx

NIFEDIPINE
(nye-<u>fed</u>-i-peen)

Purpose: treatment of hypertension and angina

• •

VERAPAMIL HCL
(ver-<u>ap</u>-a-mill)

Purpose: treatment of angina, dysrhythmias, hypertension, supraventricular tachycardia, and atrial flutter/fibrillation

ADVERSE EFFECTS

Orthostatic hypotension	Headache, dizziness	Flushing
Gingival hyperplasia	Blurred vision	Dysrhythmias
Peripheral edema	Fatigue	Sexual difficulties
Palpitations	Nausea, vomiting	Cough, fever, chills
	Rash	

NURSING CONSIDERATIONS

- PO, extended-release capsule: do not open, chew, or crush
- Take without regard to meals; onset 20 min, peak 6 hr, duration 6–8 hr
- Monitor BP when used with beta blockers
- Avoid changing positions (sitting/standing/lying) rapidly
- Do not use OTC products or alcohol unless directed by provider; limit caffeine
- Do not drink grapefruit juice; stop grapefruit juice at least 3 days prior to initiating therapy
- Protect med from light and store in dry area
- Rx

• •

ADVERSE EFFECTS

Edema	Fatigue	Impotence
Nausea, constipation	Heart failure	Nocturia
Headache	Dizziness	Rash
Drowsiness	Bruising	
	Dysrhythmias	

NURSING CONSIDERATIONS

- PO: take ac, except sustained-release, which is to be taken with food
- Do not open, chew, or crush sustained- or extended-release capsule
- Teach client how to take radial pulse and keep record of pulse rate
- Avoid hazardous activities until stabilized on med
- Do not use OTC products or alcohol unless directed by provider; limit caffeine
- Avoid grapefruit juice
- Rx

DIGOXIN
(di-<u>jox</u>-in)

Purpose: treatment of heart failure and atrial fibrillation

• •

BUMETANIDE
(byoo-<u>met</u>-a-nide)

Purpose: treatment of edema in heart failure

ADVERSE EFFECTS

Headache

Fatigue

Bradycardia

Atrial tachycardia
  (in children)

Dysrhythmias

Mental disturbances

Nausea, vomiting

Blurred vision

NURSING CONSIDERATIONS

- PO: with or without food; may crush tablets and mix with food/fluids
- Do not open, chew, or crush capsule
- Check pulse; if less than 60 bpm (adult) or 90 bpm (infant), hold med and contact provider
- Contact provider if loss of appetite, lower stomach pain, diarrhea, weakness, drowsiness, headache, blurred or yellow vision, rash, depression
- Eat a sodium-restricted and potassium-rich (bananas, orange juice) diet to keep potassium level normal
- Avoid OTC meds and herbal products; many adverse interactions may occur
- Do not stop abruptly
- Rx

• •

ADVERSE EFFECTS

Electrolyte imbalance

Hypovolemia

Hyperglycemia

Hypotension

Chest pain

Rash, pruritus

Muscle weakness

Tinnitus

Ototoxicity

Headache, dizziness

Nausea, diarrhea

Increased cholesterol

Hypokalemia

Kidney failure

Thrombocytopenia

NURSING CONSIDERATIONS

- PO: diuresis onset 30–60 min, peak 1–2 hr, duration 3–6 hr
- IM: diuresis onset 40 min, peak 1–2 hr, duration 4–6 hr
- IV: diuresis onset 5 min, peak 15–30 min, duration 3–6 hr
- May be available as generic only
- Weigh daily
- Encourage potassium-containing foods
- Monitor BUN, CBC, calcium, uric acid
- Do not take at bedtime (to prevent nocturia)
- Rx

FUROSEMIDE
(fyoo-<u>row</u>-se-mide)

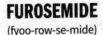

Purpose: treatment of pulmonary edema, edema in heart failure and other conditions, and hypertension

• •

TORSEMIDE
(<u>tor</u>-se-mide)

Purpose: treatment of edema in heart failure, chronic kidney failure, and liver cirrhosis; treatment of hypertension

ADVERSE EFFECTS

Orthostatic
  hypotension
Hypokalemia
Hyperglycemia
Nausea, diarrhea

Rash, pruritus
Muscle spasm
Headache, fatigue
Ototoxicity
Kidney failure

Electrolyte
imbalances
Thrombocytopenia
Photosensitivity

NURSING CONSIDERATIONS

- PO: diuresis onset 60 min, peak 1–2 hr, duration
  6–8 hr
- IV: diuresis onset 5 min, peak 30 min, duration 2 hr
- PO: take with food or milk to prevent GI upset, slightly lessened
  absorption, tablets may be crushed
- Do not give IV faster than 4 mg/min; may cause ototoxicity
- Take early in a.m. to prevent nocturia and sleeplessness
- Avoid changing positions (sitting/standing/lying) rapidly
- Rx

• •

ADVERSE EFFECTS

Hyperkalemia
Hyperglycemia
Hyperuricemia
Hypochloremic alkalosis
Hypomagnesemia
Hearing loss/deafness

Tinnitus
Hypovolemia, cardiovascular
  collapse
Dizziness
Photosensitivity

NURSING CONSIDERATIONS

- IV: give as single dose of no more than 200 mg; may not be
  given as continuous infusion
- Do not use in pregnancy or breastfeeding
- Use with caution in sulfa allergy, hypersensitivity, anuria,
  hepatic coma, severe electrolyte depletion, kidney disease
- Take in a.m. to prevent nocturia
- Check with provider before taking other meds
- Rx

SPIRONOLACTONE
(spye-ruh-no-<u>lak</u>-tone)

Purpose: treatment of edema and hypertension and of primary hyperaldosteronism

• •

CHLORTHALIDONE
(klor-<u>thal</u>-i-done)

Purpose: treatment of edema and hypertension

ADVERSE EFFECTS

Hyperkalemia

Hyponatremia

Vomiting, diarrhea

Bleeding

Rash, pruritus

Gynecomastia

Headache, confusion

Impotence

Agranulocytosis

NURSING CONSIDERATIONS

- Diuresis onset 24–48 hr, peak 48–72 hr
- Monitor electrolytes
- Weigh daily to determine fluid loss; effect of med may be decreased if used daily
- Take in a.m. to avoid interference with sleep
- Take with meals or just after to decrease gastric symptoms
- Avoid food high in potassium: oranges, bananas, salt substitutes, dried apricots, dates
- Contact provider if cramps, lethargy, menstrual abnormalities, deepening voice, breast enlargement
- Avoid potassium supplements
- Rx

• •

ADVERSE EFFECTS

Aplastic anemia

Orthostatic hypotension

Nausea, vomiting, anorexia

Urinary frequency

Electrolyte changes

Headache, dizziness

Hyperglycemia

Photosensitivity

Rash

Impotence

Hypokalemia

NURSING CONSIDERATIONS

- Diuresis onset 2 hr, peak 6 hr, duration 24–72 hr
- May be available as generic only
- Take with meals or just after to decrease gastric symptoms
- Take in a.m. to avoid interference with sleep
- Weigh daily to determine fluid loss; effect of med may decline if used daily
- Avoid changing positions (sitting/standing/lying) rapidly
- Rx

HYDROCHLOROTHIAZIDE
(hye-droe-klor-oh-<u>thye</u>-a-zide)

Purpose: treatment of edema and hypertension

• •

METOLAZONE
(meh-<u>tole</u>-a-zone)

Purpose: treatment of edema and hypertension

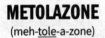

ADVERSE EFFECTS

Hypokalemia
Hyperglycemia
Nausea, vomiting, anorexia
Blurred vision
Fatigue, weakness
Confusion, esp. in older adults
Photosensitivity

Orthostatic hypotension
Electrolyte changes
Kidney failure
Aplastic anemia
Rash, urticaria
Erectile dysfunction

NURSING CONSIDERATIONS

- Diuresis onset 2 hr, peak 4 hr, duration 6–12 hr
- Take with meals or just after to decrease gastric symptoms
- Take in a.m. to avoid interference with sleep
- Hypersensitivity to sulfonamide
- Monitor electrolytes
- Rx

• •

ADVERSE EFFECTS

Dizziness, weakness, fatigue
Nausea, vomiting, anorexia

Rash
Hyperglycemia
Hypokalemia
Photosensitivity

Headache
Aplastic anemia
Impotence
Muscle cramps

NURSING CONSIDERATIONS

- Diuresis onset 1 hr, peak 2 hr, duration 12–24 hr
- Take with meals or just after to decrease gastric symptoms (slightly decreases absorption)
- Avoid changing positions (sitting/standing/lying) rapidly
- Take in a.m. to avoid interference with sleep
- Rx

KETOCONAZOLE

(key-toe-<u>kon</u>-a-zole)

Purpose: treatment of dermatological and systemic fungal infections

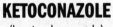

NYSTATIN

(nye-<u>stat</u>-in)

Purpose: treatment of Candida *infections*

ADVERSE EFFECTS

Photophobia   Irritation
Rash   Hepatotoxicity

NURSING CONSIDERATIONS

- PO: 200 mg daily
- Available as generic only
- Used as oral tablets or topical (cream or shampoo)
- May require several weeks or months of therapy
- Contraindicated in clients with sulfite allergy
- Take antacids 1 hr before or 2 hr after oral dose
- Do not allow shampoo to get in eyes
- Wash hands before and after use
- Rx

· ·

ADVERSE EFFECTS

GI distress, hypersensitivity
Irritation (with topical use)

NURSING CONSIDERATIONS

- Used as topical (cream, powder, ointment), oral tablets (for GI), or oral suspension
- Discontinue if redness, swelling, irritation occurs
- Encourage good oral, vaginal, skin hygiene
- Do not mix oral suspension with food
- Rx

FLUOCINONIDE
(floo-oh-<u>sin</u>-oh-nide)

Purpose: treatment of inflammation and itching caused by psoriasis, atopic dermatitis, and other skin conditions

• •

TRIAMCINOLONE ACETONIDE
(try-am-<u>sin</u>-oh-lone)

Purpose: treatment of severe inflammation caused by dermatologic disorders

ADVERSE EFFECTS

Acne
Epidermal thinning

Burning, dryness of skin
Allergic dermatitis

NURSING CONSIDERATIONS

- Topical glucocorticoid
- Apply only to affected areas; do not get in eyes
- Leave site uncovered or lightly covered
- Occlusive dressing is not recommended, systemic absorption may occur
- Do not use on weeping, denuded, or infected areas
- Avoid sunlight on affected areas
- Rx

• •

ADVERSE EFFECTS

Epidermal thinning
Burning, dryness of skin
Allergic contact dermatitis

Hypopigmentation
Hyperglycemia

NURSING CONSIDERATIONS

- Topical glucocorticoid
- Apply only to affected areas; do not get in eyes
- Leave site uncovered or lightly covered
- Occlusive dressing is not recommended; systemic absorption may occur
- Do not use on weeping, denuded, or infected areas
- Avoid sunlight on affected areas
- Rx

EXENATIDE
(ex-<u>en</u>-a-tide)

Purpose: management of type 2 diabetes mellitus

• •

GLIMEPIRIDE
(glye-<u>meh</u>-pi-ride)

Purpose: management of type 2 diabetes mellitus

ADVERSE EFFECTS

Nausea, vomiting, diarrhea
Constipation
Injection-site reactions

Hypoglycemia
Pancreatitis
Headache
Dizziness
Thyroid tumors

Anorexia, weight loss
Gastroesophageal reflux

NURSING CONSIDERATIONS

- SubQ: give extended-release product once weekly without regard to food; give immediate-release product twice daily 30 min before a meal
- Extended-release version requires reconstitution just before administration
- Both products are refrigerated before use
- Do not use in clients with severe kidney impairment or history of pancreatitis
- Routinely monitor blood glucose
- Rx

• •

ADVERSE EFFECTS

Headache
Weakness, dizziness
Drowsiness

Photosensitivity
Hepatotoxicity
Cholestatic jaundice

Increased liver enzymes

NURSING CONSIDERATIONS

- Give with a.m. meal; onset 1–1.5 hr, peak 1–3 hr, duration 10–24 hr
- Do not crush, chew, or break extended-release tablet
- Assess for symptoms of cholestatic jaundice: dark urine, pruritus, yellow sclera (rare)
- Possible cross allergy to sulfonamide
- Monitor blood glucose
- Have a quick source of sugar or glucagon emergency kit available
- Do not drink alcohol since it may produce a disulfiram reaction: nausea, headache, cramps, flushing, hypoglycemia
- Wear medical information tag
- Rx

GLIPIZIDE

(glip-i-zide)

Purpose: management of type 2 diabetes mellitus

· ·

GLYBURIDE

(glye-byoo-ride)

Purpose: management of type 2 diabetes mellitus

ADVERSE EFFECTS

Headache
Weakness, dizziness
Drowsiness

Photosensitivity
Increased liver enzymes
Cholestatic jaundice

NURSING CONSIDERATIONS

- Take with a.m. meal; onset 1–1.5 hr, peak 1–3 hr, duration 10–24 hr
- Immediate-release: take 30 min ac (absorption delayed by food)
- Assess for symptoms of cholestatic jaundice: dark urine, pruritus, yellow sclera (rare)
- May cause hemolytic anemia when used with sulfonylurea agents
- Do not drink alcohol since it can produce a disulfiram reaction: nausea, headache, cramps, flushing, hypoglycemia
- Monitor blood glucose
- Have a quick source of sugar or glucagon emergency kit available
- Wear medical information tag
- Rx

• •

ADVERSE EFFECTS

Headache
Weakness, dizziness
Photosensitivity
GI disturbances
Allergic skin reactions
Thrombocytopenia

Cholestatic jaundice
Blurred vision
Increased liver enzymes
Hepatotoxicity
Joint pain

NURSING CONSIDERATIONS

- Take with a.m. meal; onset 2–4 hr, peak 4 hr, duration 24 hr
- Assess for symptoms of cholestatic jaundice: dark urine, pruritus, yellow sclera (rare)
- Monitor blood glucose
- Have a quick source of sugar or a glucagon emergency kit available
- Wear medical information tag
- Rx

METFORMIN HCL
(met-<u>for</u>-min)

Purpose: management of type 2 diabetes mellitus

• •

PIOGLITAZONE HCL
(pye-oh-<u>glit</u>-a-zone)

Purpose: management of type 2 diabetes mellitus

ADVERSE EFFECTS

Headache

Weakness, dizziness, drowsiness

Agitation

Nausea, vomiting, diarrhea

Lactic acidosis

Thrombocytopenia

Rash

NURSING CONSIDERATIONS

- PO: twice a day with meals to decrease GI upset and provide best absorption; may also be taken as one dose
- Can crush tablets and mix with juice or soft foods for ease of swallowing
- Do not crush, chew, or break extended-release tablet
- Stop med before imaging using iodine contrast
- Be aware of signs of lactic acidosis: hyperventilation, fatigue, malaise, chills, myalgia, sleepiness
- Monitor blood glucose
- Have a quick source of sugar or glucagon emergency kit available
- Wear medical information tag
- Rx

• •

ADVERSE EFFECTS

Headache

Sinusitis

Respiratory infection

Muscle pain

MI, heart failure

Hepatotoxicity

NURSING CONSIDERATIONS

- Full therapeutic effects may require 2 or more weeks
- May exacerbate heart failure; monitor for edema and lung sounds
- Use of med for more than 1 year is associated with increased risk of bladder cancer
- Take once daily around the same time each day without regard to food
- Use in conjunction with diet and exercise regimen
- Rx

SITAGLIPTIN
(sye-ta-<u>glip</u>-tin)

Purpose: management of type 2 diabetes mellitus as monotherapy or in combination with other antidiabetic agents

INSULIN ASPART, INSULIN LISPRO
(<u>in</u>-suh-lin <u>ass</u>-part, <u>in</u>-suh-lin <u>liss</u>-pro)

Purpose: management of diabetes mellitus

ADVERSE EFFECTS

Pancreatitis
Headache
Nausea, vomiting

Acute kidney failure
Peripheral edema
Anaphylaxis

NURSING CONSIDERATIONS

- Take with or without food
- Do not split, crush, or chew tablets
- Contact provider immediately if symptoms of pancreatitis develop: persistent, severe abdominal pain with or without vomiting
- Rx

. . . .

ADVERSE EFFECTS

Hypoglycemia
Lipodystrophy
Hypokalemia

Allergic reactions
Headache
Edema

Blurred vision
Flushing

NURSING CONSIDERATIONS

- Rapid-acting insulin
- Onset 15–30 min, peak 1–3 hr, duration 3–5 hr
- May be administered IV in emergency situations under medical supervision with close blood-glucose monitoring
- Do not use inhaled form in chronic lung disease
- Available in combination with other insulin
- Provide a meal (within 5–10 min) following injection
- May be used in an external insulin pump
- May be used in children in combination with sulfonylureas
- If administered using insulin pen, read instructions carefully
- Do not mix with other insulin
- Rx

INSULIN GLARGINE
(<u>in</u>-suh-lin <u>glar</u>-jeen)

Purpose: management of diabetes mellitus

· ·

NPH INSULIN (ISOPHANE SUSPENSION)
(<u>eye</u>-soe-fain <u>in</u>-suh-lin)

Purpose: management of diabetes mellitus

ADVERSE EFFECTS

Hypoglycemia
Lipodystrophy
Allergic reactions
Headache

Edema
Blurred vision
Flushing
Hypokalemia

NURSING CONSIDERATIONS

- Long-acting insulin
- Onset 4–6 hr, no pronounced peak, duration 24 hr
- Must inject at same time each day
- Not the med of choice for diabetic ketoacidosis (use a short-acting insulin)
- Higher incidence of injection-site pain than NPH insulin
- Monitor blood glucose
- Do not administer IV or via insulin pump
- Do not mix with any other insulin
- Rx

• •

ADVERSE EFFECTS

Hypoglycemia
Lipodystrophy
Allergic reactions
Headache

Edema
Blurred vision
Flushing
Hypokalemia

NURSING CONSIDERATIONS

- Intermediate-acting insulin
- Onset 1–2 hr, peak 4–12 hr, duration 16 hr
- Comes in 100 units/milliliter vial, as well as in combination with regular insulin in a 50/50 proportion and 75/25 proportion
- Read administration instructions carefully
- Do not give IV
- Monitor blood glucose
- OTC (in some states), Rx

INSULIN, REGULAR
(<u>in</u>-suh-lin)

Purpose: management of diabetes mellitus

• •

GLUCAGON
(<u>gloo</u>-ka-gon)

Purpose: acute management of hypoglycemia, facilitation of diagnostic tests through temporary inhibition of GI tract movement

ADVERSE EFFECTS

Hypoglycemia   Hypokalemia   Blurred vision
Lipodystrophy   Headache   Flushing
Allergic reaction   Edema

NURSING CONSIDERATIONS

- Short-acting insulin
- The only insulin that can be given IV in nonemergency situations
- SubQ: onset 15–30 min, peak 30–90 min, duration 3–5 hr
- Comes in 100 units/milliliter vial
- IV: onset 10–30 min, peak 10–30 min, duration 30–60 min
- Read insulin pen instructions carefully
- May be mixed with NPH only in same syringe; draw regular insulin first
- Do not use in insulin pumps
- Monitor blood glucose
- Do not rub site after subQ injection
- OTC (in some states), Rx

• •

ADVERSE EFFECTS

Nausea, vomiting
Dizziness
Hypotension

NURSING CONSIDERATIONS

- IV: onset immediate, peak 30 min, duration 60–90 min
- SubQ: onset within 10 min, peak 13–20 min, duration 30 min
- Use reconstituted mixture within 15 min of mix
- Monitor blood glucose until client is asymptomatic
- OTC, Rx

ALUMINUM HYDROXIDE
(uh-<u>loo</u>-min-um hye-<u>drok</u>-side)

Purpose: relief of heartburn; control of hyperphosphatemia in kidney failure; adjunct therapy in ulcer treatment, GERD, and reflux esophagitis

• •

CALCIUM CARBONATE
(<u>kal</u>-see-um <u>kar</u>-buh-nate)

Purpose: relief of heartburn, calcium supplementation

ADVERSE EFFECTS

Constipation that may lead to
  impaction
Phosphate depletion

Hypomagnesemia
Hypercalciuria

NURSING CONSIDERATIONS

- PO: shake suspension well, follow with small amount of milk or water to facilitate passage; duration 20–180 min
- Contact provider if signs of GI bleeding: tarry stools, coffee-grounds vomitus
- Monitor long-term, high-dose use if on restricted sodium intake, due to high-sodium content
- If prolonged use, monitor for phosphate depletion: anorexia, malaise, muscle weakness; can also lead to resorption of calcium and bone demineralization in uremic clients
- Do not take longer than 2 weeks
- Rx

• •

ADVERSE EFFECTS

Nausea
Anorexia
Constipation

Dry mouth
Possible allergic reaction
Hypercalciuria

NURSING CONSIDERATIONS

- May decrease effect of some antibiotics and other meds due to impaired absorption, so separate administration times by 2 hr
- Do not use if ventricular fibrillation or hypercalcemia
- Use caution if taking cardiac glycoside or has sarcoidosis or kidney or cardiac disease
- Signs of hypercalcemia: nausea, vomiting, headache, confusion, anorexia
- OTC

HYOSCYAMINE
(hye-oh-<u>sye</u>-a-meen)

Purpose: treatment of peptic ulcer disease, other GI disorders, spastic disorders, IBS, and urinary incontinence

• •

LOPERAMIDE HCL
(loe-<u>pair</u>-a-mide)

Purpose: treatment of diarrhea and traveler's diarrhea

ADVERSE EFFECTS

Confusion, stimulation in older adults
Dry mouth, constipation

Urinary retention, hesitancy
Palpitations
Blurred vision, photophobia

Tachycardia
Rash
Headache
Drowsiness

NURSING CONSIDERATIONS

- PO: onset 20–30 min, duration 4–6 hr
- IM, IV, subQ: onset 2–3 min, duration 4–6 hr
- Brand names not approved by FDA
- Avoid activities requiring alertness until stabilized on med
- Avoid alcohol, CNS depressants
- Take 30–60 min ac
- Avoid antacids within 1 hr
- Rx

• •

ADVERSE EFFECTS

Nausea, vomiting
Abdominal pain/distention
Dizziness
Drowsiness

Dry mouth
Rash
Hyperglycemia
Dysrhythmias

NURSING CONSIDERATIONS

- If abdominal distention in acute ulcerative colitis, stop med
- Encourage 6–8 glasses/day of fluids
- Take with a full glass of water
- Use caution with potentially hazardous activities
- Avoid use with alcohol, CNS depressants
- Follow clear liquid or bland diet until diarrhea subsides
- Do not use OTC if fever over 101°F (38°C) or bloody diarrhea
- Use for 48 hr only
- OTC, Rx

MECLIZINE
(<u>mek</u>-li-zeen)

Purpose: management of vertigo and motion sickness

● ●

METOCLOPRAMIDE HCL
(met-oh-<u>kloe</u>-pra-mide)

Purpose: prevention of nausea and vomiting induced by chemotherapy, radiation-delayed gastric emptying, and GERD

ADVERSE EFFECTS

Drowsiness
Dizziness
Hypotension

Urinary retention
Dry mouth
Blurred vision

NURSING CONSIDERATIONS

- Duration 8–14 hr
- Take 1 hr before traveling
- Avoid activities requiring alertness
- Avoid alcohol, CNS depressants
- May give without regard to food
- OTC, Rx

• •

ADVERSE EFFECTS

Drowsiness
Restlessness, dystonia
Headache
Dry mouth

Suicidal ideation
Hypotension
Neutropenia

NURSING CONSIDERATIONS

- PO: take 30–60 min ac or procedures
- IV: inject slowly over 1–2 min; infuse over 15 min
- Used with tube feeding to decrease residual and risk of aspiration
- May cause tardive dyskinesia or neuroleptic malignant syndrome when used longer than 3 months
- Use caution with potentially hazardous activities
- Avoid alcohol, CNS depressants
- May cause depression
- Rx

K

ONDANSETRON
(on-<u>don</u>-si-tron)

Purpose: prevention of nausea and vomiting

· ·

PROMETHAZINE
(pro-<u>meth</u>-a-zeen)

*Purpose: management of motion sickness, rhinitis, allergy symptoms,
and nausea; nighttime sedation; pre- and postoperative sedation*

ADVERSE EFFECTS

Headache
Dizziness, drowsiness
GI upset

Dry mouth
Bronchospasm
Rash

NURSING CONSIDERATIONS

- Headache requiring analgesic is common
- Assess for extrapyramidal symptoms (EPS)
- Rx

• •

ADVERSE EFFECTS

Drowsiness
Dizziness
Constipation
Urinary retention
Dry mouth

Hyperglycemia
Photosensitivity
Neuroleptic
  malignant
  syndrome

Hypo/hypertension
Blurred vision
Thrombocytopenia
Respiratory
depression

NURSING CONSIDERATIONS

- PO: onset 20 min, duration 4–12 hr
- May cause severe chemical irritation and damage to tissue when used IV
- May lower seizure threshold
- May cause false results in pregnancy testing
- Take 30–60 min before traveling
- Avoid activities requiring alertness
- Avoid alcohol, CNS depressants
- Rx

SIMETHICONE
(si-<u>meth</u>-i-kone)

Purpose: reduction of pressure and bloating caused by gas in the digestive tract

• •

MISOPROSTOL
(mye-soe-<u>pross</u>-tole)

Purpose: prevention of gastric ulcers during NSAID therapy, termination of pregnancy

ADVERSE EFFECTS

Belching
Flatus

NURSING CONSIDERATIONS

- Take pc, at bedtime
- Shake suspension well before pouring
- Tablets must be chewed
- OTC, Rx

• •

ADVERSE EFFECTS

Abdominal pain	Nausea
Diarrhea	Headache
Fetal defects, pregnancy termination	Menstrual disorders

NURSING CONSIDERATIONS

- Take with meals and at bedtime
- Avoid taking magnesium antacids within 2 hr
- Notify provider if black, tarry stools, severe abdominal pain, or diarrhea
- Rx

SUCRALFATE
(soo-<u>kral</u>-fate)

Purpose: treatment of duodenal ulcers

• •

SULFASALAZINE
(sul-fuh-<u>sal</u>-a-zeen)

Purpose: treatment of ulcerative colitis and rheumatoid arthritis

ADVERSE EFFECTS

Constipation
Drowsiness, dizziness
Dry mouth

Rash, urticaria
Hyperglycemia

NURSING CONSIDERATIONS

- PO: 1 hr ac or 2 hr pc and at bedtime with full glass of water
- Do not chew or crush tablets
- Do not use antacids within 30 min of taking med
- Encourage 8–10 glasses/day of fluids
- Avoid smoking
- Not to be used for longer than 8 weeks
- Rx

• •

ADVERSE EFFECTS

Headache, confusion
Nausea, vomiting, diarrhea
Rashes
Fever
Hepatotoxicity

Kidney failure
Photosensitivity
Leukopenia
Rash, urticaria

NURSING CONSIDERATIONS

- PO: take with food to decrease GI upset
- Encourage fluids to decrease crystallization in kidneys
- May stain contact lenses, urine, and skin yellow
- Rx

PHENTERMINE
(<u>fen</u>-tur-meen)

Purpose: short-term appetite suppression

CIMETIDINE
(sye-<u>met</u>-uh-deen)

Purpose: treatment of ulcers and GERD, prevention of upper GI bleeding

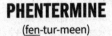

ADVERSE EFFECTS

CNS stimulation
Hyper/hypotension
Impotence
Palpitations
Drowsiness, nervousness

Dry mouth, altered taste
Bone marrow suppression
Rash, urticaria
Shortness of breath

NURSING CONSIDERATIONS

- PO, hydrochloride form: duration 4 hr
- PO, resin complex form: duration 12–14 hr
- Take 30 min ac or as a single dose before breakfast; avoid taking in late evening
- Avoid activities requiring alertness until response is known
- Avoid alcohol, CNS depressants
- Contact provider if chest pain, decreased exercise tolerance, fainting, or lower extremity swelling
- Monitor weight 3 times per week
- Rx C-IV

• •

ADVERSE EFFECTS

Diarrhea
Confusion (esp. in older adult with large doses)
Headache, dizziness
Dysrhythmias
Paralytic ileus

Agranulocytosis
Pneumonia
Rash
Impotence
Increased liver and kidney enzymes

NURSING CONSIDERATIONS

- Reduces gastric acid secretions by 50–80%
- May be taken without regard to meals
- Avoid antacids 1 hr before or after dose
- Do not use OTC meds
- OTC, Rx

FAMOTIDINE
(fuh-<u>moe</u>-ti-deen)

Purpose: treatment of ulcers, GERD, and heartburn; prevention of ulcers

• •

GLYCERIN
(glis-er-in)

Purpose: management of constipation, IBS, and diverticulosis

ADVERSE EFFECTS

Headache

Hepatitis

Dizziness

Constipation

Dysrhythmias

Taste changes

Arthralgia

Nausea, vomiting

NURSING CONSIDERATIONS

- PO: onset 60 min, peak 1–3 hr, duration 6–12 hr
- IV: onset 60 min, peak 1–4 hr, duration 12 hr
- OTC, Rx

• •

ADVERSE EFFECTS

Flatulence

Diarrhea

Abdominal disturbances

NURSING CONSIDERATIONS

- Oral, enema, or suppository
- Do not give if GI obstruction/perforation, toxic colitis, megacolon, nausea/vomiting, acute surgical abdomen
- Use with caution in rectal or anal conditions
- Infants and children are at greater risk of fluid and electrolyte disturbances
- Older adult clients are more likely to develop dependence
- OTC

LACTULOSE
(<u>lak</u>-tyoo-lose)

Purpose: relief of chronic constipation, prevention and treatment of portal-systemic encephalopathy

. . . .

POLYETHYLENE GLYCOL 3350
(pol-ee-<u>eth</u>-il-een <u>glye</u>-koll)

Purpose: short-term treatment of occasional constipation, GI bowel preparation, treatment of hyperkalemia toxicity

ADVERSE EFFECTS

Nausea, vomiting
Abdominal cramps, distention
Hypernatremia

NURSING CONSIDERATIONS

- PO: take with water or fruit juice to counteract sweet taste
- Use with caution in clients with diabetes
- Rx

• •

ADVERSE EFFECTS

Nausea	Flatulence
Abdominal bloating	Diarrhea
Cramping	

NURSING CONSIDERATIONS

- Available in different preparations: 2250, 3350, 400
- Powder form: constitute with 4–8 oz water, juice, soda, coffee, or tea
- Softens stool by increasing water absorption
- RX, OTC

PANCRELIPASE
(pan-kre-<u>lye</u>-pase)

Purpose: treatment of exocrine pancreatic secretion insufficiency and pancreatic enzyme deficiency, digestive aid for cystic fibrosis

• •

ESOMEPRAZOLE
(ess-oh-<u>meh</u>-pruh-zole)

Purpose: treatment of GERD and severe erosive esophagitis

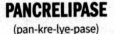

ADVERSE EFFECTS

Abdominal pain (high doses
  only)
Nausea, diarrhea
Stomach cramps

Abnormal feces
Fatigue
Hypo/hyperglycemia
Hyperuricemia

NURSING CONSIDERATIONS

- Take with 8 oz water and food, swallow right away, sit up when taking
- Do not use if sensitive or allergic to pork
- Stools will be foul-smelling and frothy
- Rx

· ·

ADVERSE EFFECTS

Headache, dizziness
Diarrhea
Nausea
Flatulence
Dry mouth

Liver failure
Rash
Cough
Heart failure
Hypoglycemia

NURSING CONSIDERATIONS

- Take at least 60 min ac
- Swallow capsules whole; do not chew
- May be taken in conjunction with antacids
- Rx

LANSOPRAZOLE
(lan-<u>soe</u>-pruh-zole)

Purpose: treatment of GERD, ulcers, and erosive esophagitis

• •

OMEPRAZOLE
(oh-<u>meh</u>-pruh-zole)

*Purpose: treatment of GERD, severe erosive esophagitis, and active
  duodenal ulcers*

ADVERSE EFFECTS

Dizziness
Constipation
Abdominal pain
Headache
Impotence

Kidney calculi
Hematuria
Hypoglycemia
Altered liver lab values

NURSING CONSIDERATIONS

- PO: take 30 min ac; capsules may be opened, sprinkled on food, and swallowed immediately
- Can use with antacids
- Report severe diarrhea
- OTC

• •

ADVERSE EFFECTS

Headache, dizziness
Nausea, vomiting, diarrhea
Flatulence
Liver failure
Rash, urticaria

Back pain
URI, cough
Electrolyte imbalances
Hypoglycemia

NURSING CONSIDERATIONS

- Take 30 min before eating
- May be taken at the same time as antacids
- Avoid activities requiring alertness
- OTC, Rx

PANTOPRAZOLE

(pan-<u>toe</u>-pruh-zole)

Purpose: treatment of GERD and ulcers, prevention of ulcers

RABEPRAZOLE

(ruh-<u>bep</u>-ruh-zole)

Purpose: treatment of GERD and ulcers

ADVERSE EFFECTS

Headache	Diarrhea	Hyponatremia
Insomnia	Pancreatitis	Hypomagnesemia
Fatigue	Rash	Muscle pain
Abdominal pain	Weight changes	

NURSING CONSIDERATIONS

- Take without regard to food
- Notify provider of black tarry stools, severe abdominal pain, or diarrhea
- Avoid alcohol, aspirin, NSAIDs
- Vitamin B_{12} deficiency may occur with long-term therapy
- Rx

• •

ADVERSE EFFECTS

Headache, dizziness	Rash	Chest pain, tachycardia
Nausea, vomiting, diarrhea	Back pain	Diarrhea
Constipation, flatulence	UTI, proteinuria	Thrombocytopenia
	Hypoglycemia	URI, cough

NURSING CONSIDERATIONS

- Take without regard to food
- Swallow tablets whole; do not crush, chew, or split tablets
- Avoid alcohol, NSAIDs, aspirin; may increase gastric upset
- Vitamin B_{12} deficiency may occur with long-term therapy
- Report severe diarrhea or black stools immediately
- Rx

TAMSULOSIN HCL
(tam-<u>soo</u>-luh-sin)

Purpose: treatment of benign prostatic hyperplasia

• •

OXYBUTYNIN CHLORIDE
(ox-ee-<u>byoo</u>-ti-nin <u>klor</u>-ide)

Purpose: prevention of spasms in neurogenic bladder, management of overactive bladder in females

ADVERSE EFFECTS

Insomnia
Nausea, vomiting, diarrhea
Blurred vision
Headache, dizziness
Increased cough

Chest pain, orthostatic
  hypertension
Floppy iris syndrome
Abnormal ejaculation, priapism

NURSING CONSIDERATIONS

- Take the same time daily, once a day, 30 min after a meal
- Do not crush, break, or chew capsules
- Avoid changing positions (lying, sitting, standing) rapidly
- Use caution in potentially hazardous activities
- Stop med before cataract surgery; may cause floppy iris syndrome
- Rx

• •

ADVERSE EFFECTS

Anxiety, restlessness
Dizziness
Seizures
Palpitations, tachycardia
Drowsiness, blurred vision
Nausea, vomiting

Anorexia
Dry mouth
Constipation
Hypertension
Impotence
Angioedema

NURSING CONSIDERATIONS

- Take without regard to meals
- Avoid alcohol, CNS depressants
- Avoid activities requiring alertness until med response is known
- Decreases ability to perspire; avoid strenuous activity in warm weather
- Rx, OTC

TOLTERODINE TARTRATE
(tol-<u>tair</u>-uh-deen)

Purpose: treatment of overactive bladder and urinary incontinence

• •

MIRABEGRON
(meer-a-<u>beg</u>-ron)

Purpose: treatment of overactive bladder

ADVERSE EFFECTS

Dry mouth
Dizziness, headache
Blurred vision
Nausea, vomiting
Dyspepsia

Constipation
UTI
Liver injury
Chest pain,
 hypertension

Anxiety
Rash, pruritus
URI, cough

NURSING CONSIDERATIONS

- Avoid alcohol during treatment
- Take without regard to meals
- Rx

• •

ADVERSE EFFECTS

Headache, dizziness
Fatigue
Hypertension
Tachycardia
Dry mouth

Constipation,
 diarrhea
Urine retention
UTI, cystitis
Flulike symptoms

Nasopharyngitis,
 sinusitis, URI
Abdominal pain
Back pain
Arthralgia

NURSING CONSIDERATIONS

- Numerous interactions with other meds
- Do not crush, chew, or cut tablets
- Avoid in severe or uncontrolled hypertension, bladder outlet obstruction, end-stage kidney disease
- Do not use in pregnancy, breastfeeding, pediatric clients
- Monitor closely for urine retention, obstruction, rash/pruritus
- Monitor liver function tests
- May increase BP or pulse; teach client how to take and monitor
- Advise client to report voiding difficulty, symptoms of bladder infection to provider
- Advise to immediately report symptoms of reaction to med
- Rx

SILDENAFIL CITRATE
(sil-<u>den</u>-a-fill <u>sih</u>-trate)

Purpose: treatment of erectile dysfunction

TADALAFIL
(tuh-<u>dal</u>-uh-fill)

Purpose: treatment of erectile dysfunction and benign prostatic hyperplasia

ADVERSE EFFECTS

Headache, flushing
Dizziness
Nasal congestion
UTI

Abnormal vision
Visual disturbance
Tinnitus, hearing loss
Rash

NURSING CONSIDERATIONS

- Take approximately 1 hr before sexual activity
- Do not use more than once a day
- Tablets may be split
- Take on empty stomach; high-fat meal reduces absorption
- Never use with nitrates; could have fatal fall in BP
- Notify provider if erection lasts longer than 4 hr
- Stop med if hearing or visual disturbances occur
- Does not protect against sexually transmitted infections
- Rx

• •

ADVERSE EFFECTS

Headache, flushing
Dyspepsia
Back pain
Tinnitus, hearing loss
Nasal congestion

Dizziness
Hypotension
UTI
Blurred vision

NURSING CONSIDERATIONS

- Take 1 hr before sexual activity
- Take at same time each day for BPH
- Avoid in clients with severe liver impairment
- Alert provider if erection lasts more than 4 hr
- Stop med if hearing or visual disturbances occur
- Alcohol intake may increase orthostatic symptoms
- Never use with nitrates; could have fatal fall in BP
- Does not protect against sexually transmitted infections
- Rx

VARDENAFIL
(var-<u>den</u>-uh-fill)

Purpose: treatment of erectile dysfunction

• •

FINASTERIDE
(fuh-<u>nas</u>-tuh-ride)

Purpose: treatment of benign prostatic hyperplasia and male pattern baldness

ADVERSE EFFECTS

Headache, dizziness
Nasal congestion
Sinusitis
Flushing
Dyspepsia, GERD

Tinnitus, hearing loss
Hypertension, chest pain
Photophobia
Arthralgia

NURSING CONSIDERATIONS

- Take 1 hr before sexual activity
- Contact provider if erection lasts over 4 hr
- Stop med if hearing or visual disturbances occur
- Never use with nitrates; could have fatal fall in BP
- Does not protect against sexually transmitted diseases
- Rx

• •

ADVERSE EFFECTS

Decreased libido
Decreased volume of ejaculate
Testicular pain
Impotence

Breast tenderness and
  enlargement
Decreased PSA levels

NURSING CONSIDERATIONS

- Full therapeutic effect may require 3–12 months
- May be taken without regard to food
- Not for use in women and children
- Pregnant women should avoid contact with crushed med or client's semen; may adversely affect developing male fetus
- Rx

NITROFURANTOIN
(<u>nye</u>-troe-fyoo-<u>ran</u>-tuh-win)

Purpose: treatment of urinary tract infection

. . . .

CHAMOMILE
(<u>kam</u>-uh-mile)

*Purpose: treatment of hay fever, inflammation, muscle spasms,
menstrual cramps, insomnia, ulcers, wounds, gastrointestinal
disorders, indigestion, rheumatic pain, mild anxiety, and hemorrhoids*

ADVERSE EFFECTS

Dizziness, headache
Nausea, vomiting, diarrhea
Abdominal pain
Tooth staining in fetus
Chills, confusion
Rash, pruritus

Chest pain
Hepatitis
Pancreatitis
Anemia
Cough, dyspnea

NURSING CONSIDERATIONS

- Take with food or milk
- Two daily doses if urine output is high or client has diabetes
- Do not break, crush, chew, or open tablets or capsules
- May turn urine rust-yellow to brown
- May cause false positive glucose in urine
- Rx

• •

ADVERSE EFFECTS

Sensitivities
Reactions with feverfew
Headache

Dizziness
Itching
Digestive disturbances

NURSING CONSIDERATIONS

- Risk of bleeding with anticoagulants
- OTC

ECHINACEA
(eh-kin-<u>ay</u>-see-uh)

Purpose: prevention and treatment of the common cold and other infections, treatment of skin wounds

• •

FEVERFEW
(<u>fee</u>-ver-fyoo)

Purpose: prophylaxis of migraine, treatment of fever and headaches

ADVERSE EFFECTS

Nausea, stomach pain
Swelling

Rash, pruritus, hives
Shortness of breath

NURSING CONSIDERATIONS

- May interfere with immunosuppressant meds and antivirals
- OTC

. . . .

ADVERSE EFFECTS

Abdominal pain
Nausea, vomiting

Digestive problems
Bloating, flatulence

NURSING CONSIDERATIONS

- Herb is well tolerated
- Decreases platelet aggregation; increased risk of bleeding with antiplatelet meds
- Contraindicated in clients with ragweed allergy
- Do not take in pregnancy; may alter uterine contractions
- OTC

GARLIC
(<u>gar</u>-lik)

Purpose: treatment of the common cold, skin wounds, high cholesterol, and high blood pressure

• •

GINGER
(<u>jin</u>-jur)

Purpose: relief of nausea, treatment of rheumatoid arthritis and osteoarthritis

ADVERSE EFFECTS

Bad breath
Body odor

Heartburn
Upset stomach

NURSING CONSIDERATIONS

- Antiplatelet effects may cause interference with warfarin
- Possible interference with immunosuppressants
- OTC

. . . .

ADVERSE EFFECTS

Mild abdominal discomfort
Heartburn

Diarrhea
Flatus

NURSING CONSIDERATIONS

- May increase risk of bleeding with anticoagulants (warfarin, heparin) and antiplatelets (aspirin, clopidogrel)
- At high doses, can interfere with cardiac, antidiabetic, or anticoagulant meds
- OTC

GINKGO
(<u>ging</u>-ko)

*Purpose: treatment of anxiety, eye diseases, peripheral artery disease,
PMS, and vertigo*

• •

GINSENG
(<u>jin</u>-seng)

*Purpose: enhancement of physical stamina, mental function, and
immune function; treatment of depression, anxiety, menopausal hot
flashes, and respiratory and cardiovascular disorders; reduction of
blood glucose and the aging process*

ADVERSE EFFECTS

Headache, dizziness
Upset stomach
Palpitations

Constipation
Allergic skin reactions

NURSING CONSIDERATIONS

- May increase risk of bleeding with anticoagulants (warfarin, heparin) and antiplatelets (aspirin, clopidogrel)
- OTC

• •

ADVERSE EFFECTS

Insomnia
Menstrual problems
Breast pain
Tachycardia

BP changes
Headache
Anorexia
Digestive problems

NURSING CONSIDERATIONS

- May interact with BP meds; monitor BP
- May affect blood glucose level; monitor clients with diabetes
- Should not be used during pregnancy
- Do not take with warfarin, MAOIs, or diabetic meds
- Long-term use may not be safe
- Stop taking 2 weeks before surgery
- OTC

ST. JOHN'S WORT

(saint <u>jahnz</u> wort)

Purpose: treatment of depression, psychiatric disorders, and IBS

• •

VALERIAN

(vuh-<u>leer</u>-ee-un)

Purpose: treatment of hay fever, inflammation, muscle spasms, menstrual disorders, insomnia, ulcers, wounds, gastrointestinal disorders, indigestion, rheumatic pain, mild anxiety, and hemorrhoids

ADVERSE EFFECTS

Weakens effects of many meds
Anxiety, irritability, restlessness
Burning or prickling sensation
Dizziness, headache
Dry mouth

Fatigue
Insomnia, vivid dreams
Photosensitivity
Hypoglycemia
GI discomfort, diarrhea

NURSING CONSIDERATIONS

- Do not use during pregnancy or breastfeeding
- May interfere with other meds: antidepressants, oral contraceptives, cyclosporine, digoxin, HIV meds, cancer meds, warfarin
- Should not be used long term
- Stop taking 2 weeks before surgery
- OTC

• •

ADVERSE EFFECTS

Sensitivities
Reactions with feverfew
Headache, dizziness

Itching
Digestive disturbances

NURSING CONSIDERATIONS

- Risk of bleeding with anticoagulants
- Increases CNS depression if used with sedatives
- OTC

ALENDRONATE
(al-en-<u>drone</u>-ate)

Purpose: treatment and prevention of osteoporosis and Paget disease

. . . .

Hormones/Synthetic Substitutes/Modifiers
Bone Resorption Inhibitors

CALCITONIN SALMON
(kal-suh-<u>toe</u>-nin <u>sam</u>-un)

Purpose: treatment of hypercalcemia, Paget disease, and osteoporosis

ADVERSE EFFECTS

Esophageal ulceration
GI distress
Musculoskeletal pain, bone
  fractures

Hypophosphatemia
Hypocalcemia
Angioedema

NURSING CONSIDERATIONS

- Onset 1 month, peak 3–6 months, duration 3 weeks to 7 months
- Take in a.m. before food or other meds with full glass of water; remain upright for 30 min
- If dose missed, skip dose; do not double dose or take later in the day
- Take with calcium and vitamin D if instructed by provider
- Rx

• •

ADVERSE EFFECTS

Headache, dizziness
Weakness
Chest pressure,
  hypertension
Nasal congestion

Nausea, vomiting,
  diarrhea
Abdominal pain
Salty taste
Diuresis, nocturia

Flushing
Myalgia, tingling of
  hands
Dyspnea,
  bronchospasms

NURSING CONSIDERATIONS

- IM/subQ: onset 15 min, peak 4 hr
- SubQ: give at bedtime to minimize nausea and vomiting, rotate injection sites
- IM: give only with epinephrine emergency meds
- Rx

RISEDRONATE
(riss-<u>ed</u>-ruh-nate)

Purpose: prevention and treatment of osteoporosis and Paget disease

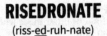

LEVOTHYROXINE
(lee-voe-thye-<u>rox</u>-een)

Purpose: management of hypothyroidism and myxedema coma

ADVERSE EFFECTS

Weakness, headache
Diarrhea, abdominal pain
Bone, back, joint pain
UTI

Fractures
Chest pain, hypertension
Hypocalcemia
Hypophosphatemia

NURSING CONSIDERATIONS

- Onset within days, peak 30 days, duration up to 16 months
- Take in a.m. before food or other meds with full glass of water; remain upright for 30 min
- Take with calcium and vitamin D if instructed by provider
- Rx

• •

ADVERSE EFFECTS

Weight loss
Dysrhythmias, tachycardia
Insomnia, irritability
Nervousness

Heat intolerance
Menstrual irregularities
Thyroid storm
Hypertension

NURSING CONSIDERATIONS

- PO: onset 24 hr
- Take at same time daily to maintain blood level; take on empty stomach
- May be toxic in large doses
- Do not switch brands unless directed by provider
- Avoid OTC meds with iodine and iodized salt, soybeans, tofu, turnips, walnuts, some seafood, some bread
- Separate antacids, iron, and calcium products by 4 hr
- Med controls symptoms and treatment is lifelong
- Rx

BUSPIRONE
(byoo-<u>spye</u>-rone)

Purpose: management of anxiety disorders

● ●

CHLORDIAZEPOXIDE
(<u>klor</u>-dye-az-uh-<u>pock</u>-side)

Purpose: management of anxiety and alcohol withdrawal

ADVERSE EFFECTS

Dizziness, headache
Insomnia, nervousness
Depression
Lightheadedness, numbness
Nausea, diarrhea, constipation
Tachycardia, palpitations

Libido changes
Hyper/hypotension
Blurred vision
Sore throat
SOB, chest congestion

NURSING CONSIDERATIONS

- Onset 7–10 days, optimum effect may take 3–4 weeks
- Available as generic only
- Use caution with activities requiring alertness until response to med is known
- Avoid alcohol, CNS depressants, grapefruit juice
- Use caution when changing positions because fainting may occur, esp. in older adults
- Drowsiness may worsen at beginning of treatment
- Rx

• •

ADVERSE EFFECTS

Dizziness
Drowsiness
Pain at IM site
Disorientation
Orthostatic hypotension

Tachycardia
Blurred vision
Decreased libido
Rash
Respiratory depression

NURSING CONSIDERATIONS

- PO: onset 30 min, peak 2 hr
- IM: onset 15–30 min; slow, erratic absorption
- IV: onset 1–5 min, duration 15–60 min
- Use caution with activities requiring alertness until response to med is known
- Abrupt stop may lead to withdrawal: insomnia, irritability, nervousness, tremors
- Avoid alcohol, CNS depressants
- Tablets may be taken with food or fluids for ease of swallowing
- Rx C-IV

DULOXETINE HCL
(doo-<u>lox</u>-uh-teen)

Purpose: treatment of major depression, neuropathic pain, anxiety, fibromyalgia, and chronic lower back pain

• •

VENLAFAXINE
(ven-luh-<u>fax</u>-een)

Purpose: treatment of depression, anxiety, and panic disorder

ADVERSE EFFECTS

Nausea, vomiting, diarrhea, constipation
Decreased appetite, stomach pain
Dry mouth
Liver failure

Increased urination, difficulty urinating
Dizziness, headache
Muscle spasms
Sexual dysfunction
Photosensitivity

Orthostatic hypotension
Palpitations
Thrombophlebitis
Hypo/hyperglycemia

NURSING CONSIDERATIONS

- Full therapeutic effect may require 4 weeks
- Taper dose before stopping
- Avoid sudden positional changes
- Avoid use with alcohol
- Use caution in potentially hazardous activities
- May increase risk of suicidal thoughts or behaviors
- Avoid aspirin, NSAIDs (increased bleeding risk)
- May cause serotonin syndrome
- Rx

. . . .

ADVERSE EFFECTS

Abnormal dreams, insomnia
Anxiety, nervousness
Headache, dizziness, weakness
Ear pain
Nausea
Bronchitis, dyspnea
Thrombocytopenia, abnormal bleeding

Sexual dysfunction
Hypertension, tachycardia
Serotonin syndrome
Photosensitivity
Hypercholesterolemia
Abnormal vision
Peripheral edema
Dysphagia

NURSING CONSIDERATIONS

- Take with food; swallow extended-release tablets whole
- Taper dose before stopping if taken longer than 6 weeks
- Avoid use with alcohol, CNS depressants for up to 1 week after end of therapy
- Use caution in potentially hazardous activities
- May increase risk of suicidal thoughts or behaviors
- Rx

CITALOPRAM
(sye-<u>tal</u>-uh-pram)

Purpose: treatment of major depression

• •

ESCITALOPRAM
(es-suh-<u>tal</u>-uh-pram)

Purpose: treatment of major depression and anxiety

ADVERSE EFFECTS

Palpitations, tachycardia
Orthostatic hypotension
Nausea, vomiting, diarrhea

Decreased appetite
Nervousness
Drowsiness
Hyponatremia
Sweating
Cough, bronchitis

Headache
Visual changes
Dry mouth
UTI
Decreased libido

NURSING CONSIDERATIONS

- Take at same time of day; therapeutic effects in up to 4 weeks
- Take at bedtime if oversedation occurs during day
- Can potentiate effects of digoxin, warfarin, diazepam
- Avoid use with alcohol, CNS depressants
- Use caution in potentially hazardous activities
- Avoid sudden positional changes
- May increase risk of suicidal thoughts or behaviors
- May cause serotonin syndrome
- Rx

• •

ADVERSE EFFECTS

GI disturbance
Fatigue, drowsiness
Decreased libido, sexual dysfunction
Dry mouth, cough, nasal congestion

Dizziness, headache
Hypokalemia
Hyponatremia
Visual disturbances
Pain, arthritis
Sweating, rash

Hot flashes, palpitations
Orthostatic hypotension
Hepatitis
Impaired platelet aggregation

NURSING CONSIDERATIONS

- Take at same time of day; therapeutic effect in up to 4 weeks
- Can potentiate effects of digoxin, warfarin, diazepam
- May require gradual reduction before stopping
- Use caution in potentially hazardous activities; avoid alcohol
- Teach client to avoid aspirin, NSAIDs (increased bleeding risk)
- May increase risk of suicidal thoughts or behaviors
- May cause serotonin syndrome
- Rx

FLUOXETINE

(floo-<u>ox</u>-uh-teen)

Purpose: treatment of major depression, OCD, bulimia, premenstrual dysphoric disorder, and panic disorder

• •

PAROXETINE

(pa-<u>rox</u>-uh-teen)

Purpose: treatment of depressive disorders, OCD, panic disorder, anxiety, PTSD, premenstrual disorders, and social anxiety

ADVERSE EFFECTS

Palpitations, hot flashes

Nausea, diarrhea, constipation

Decreased appetite

Cough, dyspnea

Nervousness, insomnia

UTI, frequency

Drowsiness

Headache

Rash, pruritus

Excessive sweating

Fatigue

Tachycardia

Visual changes

Hemorrhage

Hyponatremia

NURSING CONSIDERATIONS

- Take consistently at same time of day; full therapeutic effects may require 4 weeks
- Can potentiate effects of digoxin, warfarin, diazepam, NSAIDs, aspirin
- Avoid use with alcohol, CNS depressants
- Use caution in potentially hazardous activities
- May increase risk of suicidal thoughts or behaviors in children, adolescents, young adults
- May cause serotonin syndrome
- Rx

• •

ADVERSE EFFECTS

Palpitations, postural hypotension

Nervousness, insomnia

GI disturbance

Serotonin syndrome

Hyponatremia

Decreased appetite

Impotence

UTI

Sweating

Nasal congestion, cough

NURSING CONSIDERATIONS

- Take at same time of day; therapeutic effect in up to 4 weeks
- Decreases digoxin levels
- Take with food or milk to reduce GI symptoms
- May increase risk of bleeding
- Avoid use with alcohol, CNS depressants
- Use caution in potentially hazardous activities
- Do not discontinue abruptly
- May increase risk of suicidal thoughts or behaviors in children, adolescents, young adults
- Rx

SERTRALINE
(<u>sur</u>-truh-leen)

Purpose: treatment of major depression, OCD, PTSD, panic disorder, social anxiety disorder, and premenstrual dysphoric disorder

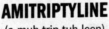

AMITRIPTYLINE
(a-muh-<u>trip</u>-tuh-leen)

Purpose: treatment of major depression

ADVERSE EFFECTS

Headache, agitation
Dizziness, confusion
Tremor
Nausea, diarrhea
Sweating

Insomnia
Dry mouth
Male sexual
  dysfunction
Palpitations

Vision
  abnormalities
SIADH
Hepatitis
Hyponatremia

NURSING CONSIDERATIONS

- Take consistently at same time of day; full therapeutic effect may require 4 weeks
- Can potentiate effects of digoxin, warfarin, diazepam, aspirin, NSAIDs
- Take with food or milk to reduce GI symptoms
- Avoid use with alcohol, CNS depressants, disulfiram
- Use caution in potentially hazardous activities
- May increase risk of suicidal thoughts or behaviors in children, adolescents, young adults
- May cause serotonin syndrome
- Rx

• •

ADVERSE EFFECTS

Sedation/drowsiness
Blurred vision,
  dry mouth,
  diaphoresis
Nausea, vomiting,
  diarrhea
Photosensitivity

Constipation,
  urinary retention
Increased appetite
Sexual dysfunction
Confusion
Tachycardia,
  dysrhythmias

Orthostatic
  hypotension
Hepatitis
Thrombocytopenia
Asthma
  exacerbation

NURSING CONSIDERATIONS

- Available as generic only
- Suicide risk high after 10–14 days due to increased energy
- Use safety precautions with hazardous activity
- Avoid alcohol, sudden positional changes
- Do not discontinue abruptly
- May increase risk of suicidal thoughts or behaviors in children, adolescents, young adults
- May cause serotonin syndrome
- Rx

DOXEPIN
(<u>dox</u>-uh-pin)

Purpose: treatment of major depression and anxiety

• •

NORTRIPTYLINE
(nor-<u>trip</u>-tuh-leen)

Purpose: treatment of major depression

ADVERSE EFFECTS

Sedation/drowsiness
Blurred vision, dry mouth,
    diaphoresis
Agranulocytosis
Sexual dysfunction
Headache, confusion
Photosensitivity

Orthostatic hypotension
Palpitations, dysrhythmias
Nausea, vomiting, diarrhea
Constipation, urinary retention
Paralytic ileus
Hepatitis
Acute kidney failure

NURSING CONSIDERATIONS

- Available as generic only
- Full therapeutic effect may require 2–3 weeks
- Suicide risk high after 10–14 days due to increased energy
- Use safety precautions with hazardous activity
- Avoid alcohol, CNS depressants, sudden positional changes
- Do not discontinue abruptly
- May increase risk of suicidal thoughts or behaviors in children, adolescents, young adults
- May worsen depression
- Rx

• •

ADVERSE EFFECTS

Sedation/
    drowsiness
Blurred vision,
    dry mouth,
    diaphoresis
Photosensitivity
Agranulocytosis

Nausea, vomiting,
    diarrhea
Constipation,
    urinary retention
Increased appetite
Sexual dysfunction
Dysrhythmias

SIADH
Acute kidney failure
Hepatitis
Orthostatic
    hypotension
Hyponatremia
Hypothyroidism

NURSING CONSIDERATIONS

- Full therapeutic effect may require 2–3 weeks
- Suicide risk high after 10–14 days due to increased energy
- Use safety precautions with hazardous activity
- Avoid alcohol, CNS depressants, sudden positional changes
- Do not discontinue abruptly
- Not approved for children
- May cause serotonin syndrome
- Rx

BUPROPION
(byoo-<u>proe</u>-pee-on)

Purpose: treatment of depression, smoking cessation

• •

MIRTAZAPINE
(mer-<u>taz</u>-uh-peen)

Purpose: treatment of depression and insomnia

ADVERSE EFFECTS

Agitation
Nausea, vomiting
Headache
Dry mouth
Weight loss/gain

Impotence
Tremor
Nervousness
Rash
Dysrhythmias

Hyper/hypotension
Blurred vision
Auditory
 disturbances

NURSING CONSIDERATIONS

- If missed dose for depression, take as soon as possible and space remaining doses at not less than 4-hr intervals
- If missed dose for smoking cessation, omit dose
- Taper dose before stopping
- Avoid use with alcohol, CNS depressants
- Use caution in potentially hazardous activities
- Avoid sudden positional changes
- May increase risk of suicidal thoughts or behaviors in children, adolescents, young adults
- Rx

● ●

ADVERSE EFFECTS

Drowsiness,
 dizziness
Increased appetite,
 weight gain
Constipation

Flulike symptoms
Dry mouth
Orthostatic
 hypotension
Palpitations

Blurred vision
Hepatitis
Kidney failure
Agranulocytosis
Photosensitivity

NURSING CONSIDERATIONS

- Therapeutic effect may take 2–3 weeks; taper dose before stopping
- Do not use within 14 days of MAOI
- Take without regard to food
- Check with provider before taking OTC cold remedy
- Avoid alcohol, CNS depressants for up to 1 week after therapy
- Use caution in potentially hazardous activities
- May increase risk of suicidal thoughts or behaviors in children, adolescents, young adults
- May cause serotonin syndrome
- Rx

TRAZODONE
(<u>traz</u>-uh-doan)

Purpose: treatment of depression

. . . .

HALOPERIDOL
(hal-oh-<u>pair</u>-i-doll)

Purpose: treatment of Tourette syndrome and schizophrenia, emergency sedation for severe agitation or delirium

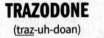

ADVERSE EFFECTS

Drowsiness	Blurred vision,	Tachycardia
Hypotension,	photosensitivity	Acute kidney failure
dizziness	Priapism	Hepatitis
Dry mouth	Constipation,	Agranulocytosis
Nausea	urinary retention	Serotonin syndrome

NURSING CONSIDERATIONS

- Therapeutic effect may take 2–3 weeks
- Available as generic only
- May increase risk of suicidal thoughts or behaviors in children, adolescents, young adults
- Taper dose before stopping
- Take at same time each day, preferably at bedtime on empty stomach
- Use caution in potentially hazardous activities
- Avoid changing positions (lying, sitting, standing) rapidly
- Avoid use with alcohol, CNS depressants
- Rx

• •

ADVERSE EFFECTS

Drowsiness	Hypotension	Hepatitis
Dizziness	EPS, confusion	GI disturbances
Dyspnea	Rash	Neuroleptic
Urinary retention	Impotence	malignancy
Tachycardia	Photosensitivity	Serotonin syndrome

NURSING CONSIDERATIONS

- PO concentrate: dilute with water, not coffee or tea
- PO: take with food or full glass of water/milk
- IM: inject slowly, deep into large muscle; have client lie down for 30 min; do not give IV
- Available as generic only
- Increased risk of death in older clients with dementia
- Avoid abrupt withdrawal; discontinue gradually
- Avoid alcohol, CNS depressants, sudden positional changes
- Use caution in potentially hazardous activities
- Rx

QUETIAPINE
(kweh-<u>tye</u>-a-peen)

Purpose: treatment of bipolar disorder, depression, and schizophrenia

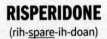

RISPERIDONE
(rih-<u>spare</u>-ih-doan)

Purpose: treatment of schizophrenia, bipolar disorder, and irritability associated with autism

ADVERSE EFFECTS

Drowsiness
Dizziness
Hyperglycemia
Nausea, anorexia
Dry mouth

Orthostatic
 hypotension
Agranulocytosis
Extrapyramidal
 symptoms (EPS)

Hyperglycemia
SIADH
Hyponatremia
Back pain

NURSING CONSIDERATIONS

- May increase the risk of suicidal thoughts or behaviors in children, adolescents, young adults
- May cause neuroleptic malignant syndrome
- Increased risk of death in older clients with dementia
- Use caution in potentially hazardous activities
- Avoid changing positions (lying/sitting/standing) rapidly
- Avoid strenuous exercise in hot weather
- Avoid use with alcohol, CNS depressants
- Avoid OTC meds unless approved by provider
- Rx

• •

ADVERSE EFFECTS

Drowsiness
Dizziness
Headache, insomnia
Constipation
Hyperglycemia
Orthostatic hypotension

EPS
Neuroleptic malignant
 syndrome
Heart failure
Neutropenia
URI

NURSING CONSIDERATIONS

- Increased risk of death in older clients with dementia
- Use caution in potentially hazardous activities
- Avoid sudden positional changes
- Avoid strenuous exercise in hot weather
- Avoid use with alcohol, CNS depressants
- Avoid OTC meds unless approved by provider
- Rx

ZIPRASIDONE
(zye-<u>praz</u>-i-doan)

Purpose: treatment of schizophrenia, acute agitation, acute psychosis, bipolar disorder, and psychotic depression

· ·

ARIPIPRAZOLE
(air-i-<u>pip</u>-ruh-zole)

Purpose: treatment of schizophrenia, bipolar disorder, and major depressive disorder

ADVERSE EFFECTS

Drowsiness
Dizziness
Abnormal vision
Headache
Anorexia, vomiting, diarrhea
Hyperglycemia

Orthostatic hypotension
Heart failure
EPS
Impotence
Decreased bone density
Rhinitis, dyspnea

NURSING CONSIDERATIONS

- May cause neuroleptic malignant syndrome
- Increased risk of death in older clients with dementia
- Use caution in potentially hazardous activities
- Avoid changing positions (lying/sitting/standing) rapidly
- Avoid strenuous exercise in hot weather
- Avoid use with alcohol, CNS depressants
- Check before taking OTC meds
- Rx

• • • • • • • • • • • • • • • • • • • •

ADVERSE EFFECTS

Headache
Insomnia
Anxiety
Cough
Weight gain
Hyperglycemia

Musculoskeletal
  pain
Nausea
Vomiting
Orthostatic
  hypotension

Neuroleptic
  malignant
  syndrome
Chest pain
Blurred vision
Rash

NURSING CONSIDERATIONS

- IM: inject deep, slowly into muscle mass; peak 1–3 hr
- PO: can take without regard to food; peak 3–5 hr
- Monitor for suicidal ideation in children, adolescents, young adults
- Increased risk of death in older clients with dementia
- Do not stop abruptly
- Rx

OLANZAPINE
(oh-<u>lan</u>-zuh-peen)

Purpose: treatment of schizophrenia and manic episodes in bipolar disorder

• •

AMPHETAMINE/DEXTROAMPHETAMINE
(am-<u>fet</u>-uh-meen / <u>decks</u>-troe-am-<u>fet</u>-uh-meen)

Purpose: treatment of ADHD and narcolepsy

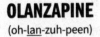

ADVERSE EFFECTS

Hostility
Headache, dizziness
Cough, pharyngitis, rhinitis
Nervousness
Joint pain
Dry mouth

Urinary retention
Insomnia
Increased appetite, weight gain
Fatigue
Impotence
Hyperlipidemia

EPS
Heart failure
Hypo/hyperglycemia
Neutropenia
Orthostatic hypotension

NURSING CONSIDERATIONS

- Initial dosage should be managed tightly
- Monitor for delirium sedation after extended-release injection
- May cause neuroleptic malignant syndrome
- Increased risk of death in older clients with dementia
- Use caution when operating equipment
- Avoid changing positions (lying/sitting/standing) rapidly
- Avoid OTC preparations unless approved by provider
- Rx

● ●

ADVERSE EFFECTS

Headache, dizziness
Weight loss
Abdominal pain
Mood changes

Tachycardia
Insomnia
Dry mouth

NURSING CONSIDERATIONS

- Take in a.m.
- High potential for abuse
- Rx C-II

LISDEXAMFETAMINE DIMESYLATE
(lis-dex-am-<u>fet</u>-a-meen dye-<u>mes</u>-i-late)

Purpose: treatment of ADHD and binge eating disorder

. . . .

METHYLPHENIDATE HCL
(meth-ill-<u>fen</u>-uh-date)

Purpose: treatment of ADD/ADHD in children over 6 years old and of narcolepsy

ADVERSE EFFECTS

Insomnia
Irritability, restlessness
Anorexia
Dry mouth

Upper abdominal pain
Tachycardia, dysrhythmias
Blurred vision, diplopia
Libido changes

NURSING CONSIDERATIONS

- For individuals age 6–64; effects have not been studied in older adults
- Interrupt therapy occasionally to determine if there is recurrence of behavioral symptoms sufficient to require continued therapy
- Children and adolescents: sudden death has been reported in clients with structural cardiac abnormalities or other serious heart problems taking CNS stimulant treatment at usual doses
- Adults: sudden death, stroke, and MI have occurred in adults taking stimulant drugs in ADHD doses
- High potential for dependency and abuse
- Rx C-II

• •

ADVERSE EFFECTS

Headache
Fever, arthralgia
Visual disturbance
Abdominal pain
Nausea, anorexia

Insomnia
Restlessness
Urticaria, rash
Leukopenia
Growth retardation

NURSING CONSIDERATIONS

- Dosage is adjusted in 18-mg increments to a maximum of 54 mg/day
- Time-released tablets/capsules should be swallowed whole, not chewed
- Do not stop abruptly; taper over several weeks
- Monitor for adverse psychiatric symptoms
- High potential for dependency and abuse
- Avoid alcohol, caffeine, OTC preparations
- Rx C-II

ALPRAZOLAM

(al-<u>praz</u>-uh-lam)

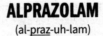

Purpose: management of anxiety and panic disorder

CLONAZEPAM

(kloe-<u>naz</u>-uh-pam)

Purpose: management of seizures and panic disorder

ADVERSE EFFECTS

Dizziness, drowsiness

Orthostatic hypotension

Blurred vision

Memory impairment

Increased appetite

Suicidal ideation

Constipation, dry mouth

Decreased libido

NURSING CONSIDERATIONS

- Onset 30 min, peak 1–2 hr, duration 4–6 hr
- Full therapeutic response takes 2–3 days
- Drowsiness may worsen at beginning of treatment
- Do not stop med abruptly; may cause seizures
- Monitor for respiratory depression
- Memory impairment is a sign of long-term use
- May be taken with food
- May be habit-forming; do not take for longer than 4 months unless directed
- Rx C-IV

• •

ADVERSE EFFECTS

Drowsiness, dizziness

Behavioral changes

Poor coordination

Palpitations, tachycardia

Blurred vision

Increased salivation

Nausea, constipation

Dysuria

Libido changes

Thrombocytopenia

Respiratory depression

Rash

Muscle weakness

NURSING CONSIDERATIONS

- May take with food or milk to decrease GI symptoms
- Do not discontinue abruptly; seizures may increase
- Avoid alcohol, CNS depressants
- Report signs of toxicity: bone marrow suppression, nausea, vomiting, ataxia, diplopia, cardiovascular collapse
- May increase risk of suicidal thoughts
- Wear medical information tag
- Rx C-IV

DIAZEPAM
(dye-<u>az</u>-uh-pam)

Purpose: management of anxiety, alcohol withdrawal, and seizure disorders; relaxation of skeletal muscle; preoperative sedation

• •

LORAZEPAM
(lor-<u>az</u>-uh-pam)

Purpose: management of anxiety and irritability in psychiatric disorders, treatment of insomnia, adjunct therapy for endoscopic procedures, relief of preoperative anxiety

217

ADVERSE EFFECTS

Drowsiness, fatigue, ataxia

Paradoxic anxiety, esp. in
older adults

Orthostatic hypotension

Blurred vision

Neutropenia

Constipation, dry mouth

Respiratory depression

NURSING CONSIDERATIONS

- PO: may be taken with food, onset 30 min, peak 2 hr
- IM: inject deep, slowly into large muscle mass; onset 15–30 min, duration 60–90 min; slow and erratic absorption
- IV: infuse into large vein; onset immediate, duration 15–60 min; push doses should not exceed 5 mg/min; have resuscitation equipment available
- Smoking may decrease effectiveness
- Avoid use with alcohol, CNS depressants
- May be habit-forming if used longer than 4 months
- Do not discontinue abruptly after long-term use
- Rx C-IV

. . . .

ADVERSE EFFECTS

Dizziness, drowsiness

Orthostatic hypotension

Blurred vision

Weakness, headache

Disorientation

Constipation, dry mouth

Rash, dermatitis

Acidosis

NURSING CONSIDERATIONS

- PO: onset 1 hr, peak 2 hr
- IM: onset 15–30 min, peak 60–90 min
- IV: onset 5–15 min, peak 60–90 min
- Drowsiness may worsen at beginning of treatment
- Do not stop med abruptly after long-term use
- Monitor for respiratory depression
- May be taken with food
- May be habit-forming; do not take for longer than 4 months unless directed
- Avoid alcohol, CNS depressants
- Rx C

TEMAZEPAM
(tem-<u>az</u>-uh-pam)

Purpose: short-term treatment of insomnia

. . . .

Mental Health Medications
Bipolar Agents

LITHIUM
(<u>lith</u>-ee-um)

Purpose: management of manic phase in bipolar disorder, prevention of bipolar manic-depressive psychosis

ADVERSE EFFECTS

Drowsiness

Dizziness, headache

Lethargy, fatigue

Weakness

Euphoria

Chest pain, hypotension

Blurred vision

Nausea, vomiting, anorexia

NURSING CONSIDERATIONS

- Take without regard to food
- Not intended for use for more than 10 days
- Should be avoided in clients under the age of 18
- Monitor for respiratory depression
- Increases the effect of CNS depressants
- Avoid alcohol while taking this medication
- "Sleep driving" may occur, esp. if taken with alcohol or CNS depressants
- Rx C-IV

• •

ADVERSE EFFECTS

Signs of toxicity: vomiting,
diarrhea, drowsiness, muscular
weakness, ataxia

Dizziness, headache

Impaired vision

Fine hand tremors

Reversible leukocytosis

Dry mouth, anorexia

Hypotension, dysrhythmias

Polyuria, proteinuria

Hyponatremia

Hypo/hyperthyroidism

NURSING CONSIDERATIONS

- Onset of therapeutic effects in 1–2 weeks
- Check serum levels twice weekly during treatment, q 2–3 months on maintenance; draw blood in a.m. prior to dose
- Target serum levels: treatment = 0.5 to 1.5 mEq/L, maintenance = 0.6–1.2 mEq/L
- Take with meals to avoid GI upset
- Use caution in potentially hazardous activities
- Dose reduced during depressive stages of illness
- Encourage 10–12 glasses/day of fluids, 6–10 g/day salt intake
- Rx

ZALEPLON
(<u>zall</u>-uh-plon)

Purpose: short-term treatment of insomnia

· ·

ZOLPIDEM TARTRATE
(<u>zol</u>-pi-dem)

Purpose: short-term treatment of insomnia

ADVERSE EFFECTS

Headache, tremors
Myalgia
Dizziness, confusion

Bronchitis
Dyspepsia, dry mouth
Eye pain, vision change

NURSING CONSIDERATIONS

- Because of rapid onset, clients should take immediately before bedtime
- Older adult clients generally benefit the most
- May be habit-forming
- May cause complex sleep behaviors causing injury or death
- Avoid alcohol while using this med
- Rx C-IV

• •

ADVERSE EFFECTS

Headache
Drowsiness
Dizziness
Nausea

"Drugged" feeling
Abnormal thinking
Leukopenia
Myalgia

NURSING CONSIDERATIONS

- Reduce dose in client using a CNS depressant, to avoid addiction
- Adverse effects increase with prolonged usage
- May cause complex sleep behaviors causing injury or death
- May worsen depression
- Monitor for suicidal thoughts or behavior
- Rx C-IV

ALLOPURINOL
(al-oh-<u>pure</u>-i-nole)

Purpose: treatment of gout and uric acid calculi, management of chemotherapy-induced hyperuricemia in clients with leukemia or lymphoma

. . . .

COLCHICINE
(<u>kol</u>-chi-seen)

Purpose: prevention and treatment of gouty arthritis, treatment of gout and Mediterranean fever

ADVERSE EFFECTS

GI upset
Rash
Malaise

NURSING CONSIDERATIONS

- Full therapeutic effect may require several months
- Check CBC, kidney and liver function tests before treatment
- Initial therapy can increase attacks of gout
- Take with food
- Encourage 10–12 glasses/day of fluids
- Avoid alcohol, organ meats, gravy, legumes
- Rx

• •

ADVERSE EFFECTS

Signs of toxicity: abdominal
  cramp, weakness, nausea,
  vomiting
Agranulocytosis

Hematuria
Kidney damage
Chills, dermatitis
Diarrhea

NURSING CONSIDERATIONS

- IV: infuse slowly; do not administer IM/subQ
- Has analgesic, anti-inflammatory effects
- May be taken without regard to meals
- Encourage 10–12 glasses/day of fluids
- Avoid grapefruit products, alcohol, organ meats, gravy, legumes
- Rx

PROBENECID
(proe-<u>ben</u>-uh-sid)

*Purpose: treatment of hyperuricemia in gout and gouty arthritis,
adjunct to penicillin treatment*

. . . .

ADALIMUMAB
(ay-duh-<u>lim</u>-yoo-mab)

*Purpose: management of rheumatoid arthritis, psoriatic arthritis,
Crohn disease, plaque psoriasis, ankylosing spondylitis, and
ulcerative colitis*

ADVERSE EFFECTS

Nausea
Anorexia
Apnea
Hyperglycemia
Skin rash
Hemolytic anemia

Drowsiness, headache
Hypokalemia
Bradycardia
Liver necrosis
Nephrotic syndrome

NURSING CONSIDERATIONS

- Available as generic only
- Give with milk, food, and antacids
- Encourage 8–10 glasses/day of fluids
- Avoid alcohol, organ meats, gravy, legumes
- Avoid aspirin-containing products; may take acetaminophen
- Rx

. . . .

ADVERSE EFFECTS

Headache
Hypertension, heart failure
Sinusitis
GI bleeding
Abdominal pain, nausea
Liver damage

Leukopenia
Flulike symptoms
Increased cancer risk
UTI
URI, bronchitis

NURSING CONSIDERATIONS

- Screen for TB before starting treatment
- Treat latent tuberculosis before initiating therapy
- Increased risk for serious infections
- May reactivate hepatitis B in chronic carriers
- Rx

DICLOFENAC NA
(dye-<u>kloe</u>-fen-ak)

Purpose: management of rheumatoid arthritis, osteoarthritis, and dysmenorrhea

• •

ETANERCEPT
(eh-<u>tan</u>-ur-sept)

Purpose: management of acute chronic rheumatoid arthritis, ankylosing spondylitis, and plaque psoriasis

ADVERSE EFFECTS

Dizziness, drowsiness
Blood dyscrasias
Headache
Nephrotoxicity
Hepatotoxicity
GI distress, bleeding, or ulcer
Rash

Heart failure
Dysrhythmias
MI/stroke
Hearing loss, blurred vision
Photosensitivity
Hyperglycemia
Thromboembolism

NURSING CONSIDERATIONS

- Use with NSAIDs increases anticoagulant effects
- Do not use before or after CABG surgery
- Increased infection risk
- PO: take with full glass of water and food and remain upright for 30 min
- If dose missed, take within 2 hr
- Rx

• •

ADVERSE EFFECTS

Headache
Dizziness
Abdominal pain

Dyspepsia
Heart failure
Hepatitis

Anemia, leukopenia
URI, cough

NURSING CONSIDERATIONS

- Instruct client or caregiver to administer subQ injection
- Do not take live viruses during treatment
- Increased risk for cancer development
- Increased risk of serious infection
- Must be continued for prescribed time to be effective
- Rx

INDOMETHACIN
(in-doe-<u>meth</u>-a-sin)

Purpose: treatment of rheumatoid arthritis, osteoarthritis, bursitis, tendinitis, acute gouty arthritis, and ankylosing spondylitis

· ·

PIROXICAM
(peer-<u>ox</u>-i-kam)

Purpose: relief of mild to moderate pain in osteoarthritis and rheumatoid arthritis

ADVERSE EFFECTS

Peptic ulcer	Drowsiness	GI bleeding
Dizziness, headache	Nausea,	Hepatitis
Blurred vision	constipation	Blood dyscrasias
Tinnitus	Dysrhythmias	Nephrotoxicity
Hypertension	MI/stroke	Thrombosis

NURSING CONSIDERATIONS

- PO: take with food/milk, encourage upright position for 15–30 min
- Do not give after CABG surgery
- Use caution with potentially hazardous activities
- Avoid use with alcohol, aspirin, other NSAIDs
- Rx

• •

ADVERSE EFFECTS

Drowsiness, dizziness	Exacerbation of angina
Nausea, vomiting	Anemia, leukopenia
Blurred vision, tinnitus	Photosensitivity
GI disturbance, bleeding, or ulcer	Hypo/hyperglycemia
	Kidney failure
Rash	Bronchospasms

NURSING CONSIDERATIONS

- PO: with food to decrease GI upset; on empty stomach to increase absorption
- Do not give after CABG surgery
- Increased risk for MI or stroke
- Take at same time every day
- Full therapeutic effect may take up to 1 month for arthritis
- Avoid concurrent use of aspirin, OTC meds, alcohol
- Rx

BACLOFEN
(<u>bak</u>-loe-fen)

Purpose: reduction of spasticity in spinal cord injuries and multiple sclerosis

• •

CARISOPRODOL
(kar-eye-soe-<u>proe</u>-dole)

Purpose: relief of pain and stiffness in musculoskeletal disorders

ADVERSE EFFECTS

Drowsiness
Dizziness
Weakness, fatigue
Confusion
Nausea, vomiting
Headache

Seizures
Hypotension
Chest pain, palpitations
Blurred vision
Respiratory failure
Urinary frequency

NURSING CONSIDERATIONS

- Increased risk of seizures in clients with seizure disorder
- Take with food to decrease GI symptoms
- Avoid alcohol, CNS depressants
- Do not discontinue abruptly, unless severe adverse reaction; taper over 1–2 weeks; may precipitate hallucinations, tachycardia, rebound spasticity
- Rx

• •

ADVERSE EFFECTS

Drowsiness
Headache
Insomnia
Dizziness

Nausea
Postural
 hypotension
Diplopia

Asthma attacks
Eosinophilia
Rash

NURSING CONSIDERATIONS

- PO: onset 30 min, peak 4 hr, duration 4–6 hr
- Avoid alcohol, CNS depressants (including OTC cold or allergy meds)
- Avoid activities requiring alertness until effects of med are known
- May cause dependence; use for short term (2–3 weeks)
- Rx C-IV

CYCLOBENZAPRINE
(sye-kloe-<u>ben</u>-za-preen)

Purpose: relief of muscle spasms and pain in musculoskeletal conditions

• •

METHOCARBAMOL
(meth-oh-<u>kar</u>-ba-mole)

*Purpose: relief of pain associated with musculoskeletal disorders,
adjunct in management of neuromuscular manifestations of tetanus*

ADVERSE EFFECTS

Drowsiness	Constipation	Dysrhythmias
Dizziness	Headache	Diplopia
Fatigue	Hepatitis	Libido changes
Rash	Postural	Respiratory
Dry mouth	hypotension	depression

NURSING CONSIDERATIONS

- Give with food to decrease GI upset
- Avoid alcohol, CNS depressants, OTC cold and allergy meds
- Avoid activities requiring alertness until effects of med are known
- Do not discontinue abruptly; taper over 1–2 weeks
- Rx

• •

ADVERSE EFFECTS

Drowsiness	Dizziness	Urticaria
Lightheadedness	Nausea	Blurred vision
Hypotension	Metallic taste	

NURSING CONSIDERATIONS

- IM: inject deep into muscle of buttock, rotate sites
- NG tube: crush tablets into fluid
- PO: take with food or milk
- Monitor IV sites carefully for extravasation
- Urine may turn green, black, or brown
- Avoid alcohol, CNS depressants, including OTC cold or allergy meds
- Avoid activities requiring alertness until effects of med are known
- Rx

BENZTROPINE
(<u>benz</u>-troe-peen)

Purpose: treatment of Parkinson symptoms, EPS associated with neuroleptic meds, and acute dystonic reactions

· ·

CARBIDOPA/LEVODOPA
(kar-bih-<u>doe</u>-pa/<u>leev</u>-oe-doe-pa)

Purpose: treatment of Parkinson disease and syndrome

ADVERSE EFFECTS

Dry mouth
Constipation
Weakness
Tardive dyskinesia
Anxiety, irritability
Dizziness, confusion

Palpitations
Hypotension
Photophobia
Urinary retention
Hyperthermia

NURSING CONSIDERATIONS

- IM/IV: onset 15 min, duration 6–10 hr
- PO: onset 1 hr, duration 6–10 hr
- Available as generic only
- Tablets may be crushed and mixed with food
- Avoid hazardous activities until stabilized on med
- Change positions slowly
- Avoid alcohol, antihistamines unless directed by provider
- Taper med over a week, or withdrawal symptoms: EPS, tremors, insomnia, tachycardia, restlessness
- Rx

• •

ADVERSE EFFECTS

Twitching
Headache, dizziness
Mental changes: confusion, agitation, mood alterations
Dark urine/sweat
Cardiac dysrhythmias

Orthostatic hypotension
Blurred vision
Nausea, vomiting
Hemolytic anemia
Rash
Increased liver function tests

NURSING CONSIDERATIONS

- Full therapeutic effect may take several months
- Take without food, ac; decreased effect with protein
- Change positions slowly
- May cause false positive for urine ketones
- May cause neuroleptic malignant syndrome
- Rx

SELEGILINE
(se-<u>leh</u>-ji-leen)

Purpose: management of Parkinson disease in clients being treated with levodopa/carbidopa

• •

DONEPEZIL
(doe-<u>nep</u>-uh-zill)

Purpose: management of dementia in Alzheimer disease

ADVERSE EFFECTS

Dizziness
Photosensitivity
Nausea, diarrhea
Headache

Shortness of breath
Insomnia
Orthostatic
  hypotension

Dysrhythmias
Sexual dysfunction
Diplopia

NURSING CONSIDERATIONS

- Do not use with tricyclics or opioids
- Monitor for signs of toxicity: twitching, eye spasms
- Do not stop abruptly; parkinsonian crisis may occur
- Do not use transdermal patch for children under age 12
- Transdermal may increase risk of suicide in children, adolescents, young adults
- Avoid foods high in tyramine (cheese, pickled products), alcohol, large amounts of caffeine
- Rx

• •

ADVERSE EFFECTS

Nausea, vomiting, diarrhea
Headache, dizziness
Fatigue
Cardiac dysrhythmias
Insomnia
Seizures
Rash

Dark urine/sweat
Mental changes
Hypo/hypertension
GI bleeding
Hyperlipidemia
UTI
URI

NURSING CONSIDERATIONS

- Med does not cure, but stabilizes or relieves symptoms
- Take at regular intervals
- Take between meals or may be given with meals to decrease GI upset
- Rx

GALANTAMINE, RIVASTIGMINE
(ga-<u>lan</u>-ta-meen, ri-va-<u>stig</u>-meen)

Purpose: treatment of dementia in mild to moderate Alzheimer disease

· ·

MEMANTINE HCL
(<u>mem</u>-an-teen)

Purpose: treatment of moderate to severe dementia in Alzheimer disease

ADVERSE EFFECTS

Nausea
Vomiting
Diarrhea
URI

Anemia
Bradycardia
Tremors, insomnia

NURSING CONSIDERATIONS

- Both meds are cholinesterase inhibitors, which increase acetylcholine in the brain, potentially reducing symptoms of dementia
- Meds do not cure, but stabilize or relieve symptoms
- Use with caution in clients with liver, bladder, or kidney disease
- Rx

• •

ADVERSE EFFECTS

Headache
Constipation
Confusion
Dizziness
Heart failure

Hypertension
Anemia
Back pain
Cough, dyspnea

NURSING CONSIDERATIONS

- Capsules can be opened and contents sprinkled on applesauce for clients who have difficulty swallowing pills
- Use with caution in clients with liver, bladder, or kidney disease
- Rx

ZOLMITRIPTAN
(zole-mih-<u>trip</u>-tan)

Purpose: acute treatment of migraines

. . . .

DORZOLAMIDE HCL
(dor-<u>zoh</u>-la-mide)

Purpose: treatment of glaucoma and ocular hypertension

ADVERSE EFFECTS

Weakness, neck stiffness
Tingling, hot sensation,
  burning, feeling of pressure,
  tightness
Numbness, dizziness, sedation

Palpitations, chest pain
Abdominal discomfort
Dyspepsia
Dry mouth

NURSING CONSIDERATIONS

- Take as soon as symptoms occur
- Avoid foods high in tyramine (cheese, pickled products), alcohol, large amounts of caffeine
- May cause serotonin syndrome when used with antidepression medication
- Rx

• •

ADVERSE EFFECTS

Ocular burning, stinging,
  discomfort
Blurred vision, tearing, dryness

Photophobia
Bitter taste in mouth

NURSING CONSIDERATIONS

- Drug is a sulfonamide; although given topically, it can be absorbed systemically
- Wash hands before and after instillation
- Do not touch tip of dropper to eye or body
- Do not wear contact lenses during instillation
- Rx

LATANOPROST
(luh-<u>tan</u>-uh-prahst)

Purpose: treatment of glaucoma and ocular hypertension

• •

TRAVOPROST
(<u>trav</u>-oh-prahst)

Purpose: treatment of glaucoma and ocular hypertension

ADVERSE EFFECTS

Iris color change

Visual disturbances

Foreign body sensation

Eye discomfort, pain

Angina

NURSING CONSIDERATIONS

- For clients unresponsive to other IOP-lowering meds
- Wash hands before and after instillation
- Do not touch tip of dropper to eye or body
- Remove contact lenses to give med; can reinsert in 15 min
- Rx

• •

ADVERSE EFFECTS

Ocular hyperemia

Decreased visual acuity

Eye discomfort or pain

Foreign-body sensation

Eye pruritus

NURSING CONSIDERATIONS

- For clients intolerant of or unresponsive to other IOP-lowering medications
- Wash hands before and after instillation
- Do not touch tip of dropper to eye or body
- Place pressure on tear ducts for 1 min to avoid systemic absorption
- Potential for increased brown pigmentation of iris, eyelid skin darkening, changes in eyelashes; important if only one eye is being treated
- Remove contact lenses to give med; can reinsert in 15 min
- Discard med 6 months after opening
- Rx

LEVOBUNOLOL
(lee-voe-<u>byoo</u>-no-lole)

Purpose: treatment of glaucoma and ocular hypertension

• •

TIMOLOL
(<u>tim</u>-oh-lole)

Purpose: treatment of glaucoma and ocular hypertension

ADVERSE EFFECTS

Hypotension
Transient eye stinging and
  burning

Palpitations
Insomnia, headache
Bronchospasm

NURSING CONSIDERATIONS

- Wash hands before and after instillation
- Do not touch tip of dropper to eye or body
- Place pressure on tear ducts for 1 min to decrease systemic absorption
- Report shortness of breath, chest pain, or heart irregularity
- Rx

• •

ADVERSE EFFECTS

Fatigue
Weakness
Hypotension
Burning and stinging of eye

Palpitations
Heart failure
Bronchospasm

NURSING CONSIDERATIONS

- Wash hands before and after instillation
- Avoid touching eye or body with med container
- Place pressure on tear ducts for 1 min to decrease systemic absorption
- Rx

BRIMONIDINE TARTRATE
(brih-<u>moh</u>-nih-deen)

Purpose: treatment of glaucoma and ocular hypertension

• •

TOBRAMYCIN/DEXAMETHASONE
(toe-bruh-<u>mye</u>-sin/dex-uh-<u>meth</u>-uh-sone)

Purpose: treatment of conjunctivitis

ADVERSE EFFECTS

Pruritus

Cough, dyspnea

Fatigue

Hypertension

Visual disturbance

Eye stinging/burning

Photophobia

Hypercholesterolemia

NURSING CONSIDERATIONS

- Monitor intraocular pressure: may reverse after 1 month of therapy
- Wash hands before and after instillation
- Wait 15 min after use to wear soft contact lenses
- Use caution with hazardous activities due to decreased mental alertness
- Avoid alcohol
- Rx

• •

ADVERSE EFFECT

Ocular irritation

NURSING CONSIDERATIONS

- Wash hands before and after instillation
- Do not touch tip of dropper to eye or body
- Do not wear contact lenses while using this med
- Rx

ANTIPYRINE/BENZOCAINE/GLYCERIN OTIC SOLUTION
(an-tee-<u>pye</u>-reen/<u>ben</u>-zoe-kane/<u>gli</u>-sa-rin <u>oh</u>-tik)

Purpose: relief of pain and inflammation in ear

• •

HYDROCORTISONE/NEOMYCIN/ POLYMYXIN OTIC
(hye-droe-<u>kor</u>-tir-sone/nee-uh-<u>mye</u>-sin/pol-i-<u>mix</u>-in <u>oh</u>-tik)

Purpose: treatment of ear infections

ADVERSE EFFECTS

Allergic reaction: rash, difficulty breathing

NURSING CONSIDERATIONS

- Brand names not approved by FDA
- Suspension: shake well (also comes in solution)
- Can warm up with hands for client's comfort
- Warn client not to touch ear with dropper
- Warn client that med is for use in ears only
- Do not get in eyes, nose, or mouth
- May place cotton plug moistened with med in ear canal
- Do not rinse dropper
- Rx

• •

ADVERSE EFFECTS

Allergic reaction: rash, difficulty breathing
Burning

NURSING CONSIDERATIONS

- Warn client not to touch ear with dropper
- Explain med is for use in ears only
- Possible cross allergy with kanamycin, paromomycin, streptomycin, gentamicin
- Rx

MONTELUKAST
(mon-te-<u>lew</u>-kast)

Purpose: prophylaxis and treatment of asthma and seasonal allergic rhinitis

• •

THEOPHYLLINE
(thee-<u>off</u>-i-lin)

Purpose: treatment of bronchial asthma, bronchospasm of chronic bronchitis, and emphysema

ADVERSE EFFECTS

Dizziness
Headache
Cough
GI upset

Thrombocytopenia
Pancreatitis
Nasal congestion
Muscle cramps

NURSING CONSIDERATIONS

- Full therapeutic effect may take several weeks
- Do not use to treat acute symptoms; use a rapid-acting bronchodilator
- Notify provider of wheezing, respiratory distress
- May increase risk of neuropsychiatric events including hallucination, aggression, anxiousness, suicidal behavior and thoughts, tremor
- Rx

• •

ADVERSE EFFECTS

Restlessness
Palpitations, sinus
tachycardia
Dizziness

Anorexia
Vomiting
Headache
Insomnia

SIADH
Flushing
Hyperglycemia
Tachypnea

NURSING CONSIDERATIONS

- PO: peak 2 hr; take with full glass of water; best on empty stomach
- Check all OTC and other meds for ephedrine before taking with this med
- Avoid alcohol, caffeine, smoking
- Avoid activities requiring alertness until response to med is known
- Contact provider if toxicity: nausea, vomiting, anxiety, insomnia, convulsions
- Drink 8–10 glasses/day of fluids
- Rx

TIOTROPIUM
(tye-oh-<u>troe</u>-pee-um)

Purpose: prevention of bronchial swelling and bronchospasms associated with COPD

• •

BENZONATATE
(ben-<u>zoe</u>-na-tate)

Purpose: treatment of nonproductive cough

ADVERSE EFFECTS

Oral thrush
Vomiting, abdominal pain
Skeletal pain
Pharyngitis
Cough, URI

Depression
Paresthesia
Chest pain, increased heart rate
Dry mouth
Urinary difficulty

NURSING CONSIDERATIONS

- Oral inhalation: onset 30 min, peak 2 hr, duration 24 hr
- Do not use as a rescue inhaler (delayed onset, long duration of action)
- Take once daily
- Teach how to correctly use inhaler: insert dry powder capsule into inhaler device just before inhalation; do not swallow capsules; rinse mouth with water after inhalation (decreases adverse effects)
- Rx

• •

ADVERSE EFFECTS

Dizziness
Drowsiness
Rash

Sedation, headache
Nausea
Constipation

NURSING CONSIDERATIONS

- PO: onset 15–20 min, duration 3–8 hr
- Capsules should be swallowed whole; do not chew, because release of med may cause local anesthetic effect and choking
- Avoid activities requiring alertness until response to med is known
- Rx

IPRATROPIUM
(eye-pra-<u>troe</u>-pee-um)

Purpose: treatment of bronchospasms, COPD, and rhinorrhea

• •

ALBUTEROL SULFATE
(al-<u>byoo</u>-ter-ol)

Purpose: prevention of exercise-induced asthma, acute bronchospasm, bronchitis, and emphysema

ADVERSE EFFECTS

Nervousness   Dry mouth   Blurred vision
Nausea, cramps   Palpitations   Headache

NURSING CONSIDERATIONS

- Not for acute bronchospasm needing rapid response
- Teach use of metered-dose inhaler: inhale, hold breath, exhale slowly
- Can use with spacer
- Don't mix in nebulizer with cromolyn sodium
- Assess for hypersensitivity, including soy products, atropine, peanuts
- Encourage 10–12 glasses/day of fluids
- Avoid OTC cough/hay-fever meds
- Use caution with hazardous activities
- Rx

• •

ADVERSE EFFECTS

Tremors, anxiety   Dry nose
Headache   Restlessness, insomnia
Tachycardia, palpitations   Hypo/hypertension
Hypokalemia   Muscle cramps
Heartburn, nausea   Paradoxical bronchospasms

NURSING CONSIDERATIONS

- Monitor for toxicity
- Teach client how to correctly use inhaler
- Can use with spacer
- Rx

BUDESONIDE/FORMOTEROL
(byoo-<u>dess</u>-oh-nide/for-<u>mot</u>-ur-all)

Purpose: prevention of bronchospasm in asthma and COPD

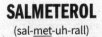

SALMETEROL
(sal-<u>met</u>-uh-rall)

Purpose: prevention of exercise-induced bronchospasms, treatment of COPD and asthma

ADVERSE EFFECTS

Thrush
Throat irritation
Vomiting,
  abdominal pain

Flulike symptoms
Back pain
Headache

Respiratory
  infection

NURSING CONSIDERATIONS

- Not for bronchospasms needing rapid response
- Rinse mouth with water after each use
- Teach proper use of inhaler
- Rx

- -

ADVERSE EFFECTS

Headache
Tremors, anxiety
Throat irritation
Myalgia

Nausea, vomiting
Cough
Palpitation,
  dysrhythmias

Hypo/hypertension
Dry nose
Paradoxical
  bronchospasm

NURSING CONSIDERATIONS

- Teach client inhaler setup and use
- May increase risk of death from asthma
- Should be used with long-term asthma-control medication
- Do not use to treat acute symptoms; do not use as a rapid-acting bronchodilator
- Contact provider if using more than 4 inhalations of a rapid-acting bronchodilator for 2 or more consecutive days
- Rx

TERBUTALINE SULFATE
(ter-<u>byoo</u>-ta-leen)

Purpose: treatment of bronchospasms, suppression of preterm labor

• •

GUAIFENESIN
(gwye-<u>fen</u>-uh-sin)

Purpose: relief of chest congestion by loosening mucus and bronchial secretions

ADVERSE EFFECTS

Nervousness

Restlessness

Tremor

Palpations, dysrhythmias

Headache

Hypokalemia

Hyperglycemia

Paradoxical bronchospasms

NURSING CONSIDERATIONS

- Available as generic only
- Inhalation and subQ used for short-term control; PO as long-term
- Only short-term use for tocolysis
- Do not use to prevent preterm labor or birth
- PO: take with food to decrease GI upset
- Contact provider if unrelieved shortness of breath
- Do not use OTC meds without contacting provider
- Rx

• •

ADVERSE EFFECTS

Nausea

Headache

Dizziness

Anorexia

NURSING CONSIDERATIONS

- Do not crush pills
- Take with full glass of water
- Increase fluid intake
- OTC, Rx

CROMOLYN SODIUM
(<u>kroe</u>-moe-lin)

Purpose: prophylaxis and treatment of allergic rhinitis and bronchial asthma

· ·

DISULFIRAM
(dye-<u>sul</u>-fih-ram)

Purpose: treatment of alcoholism

ADVERSE EFFECTS

Nasal burning and irritation
Headache
Dry mouth

Rash
Bronchospasm

NURSING CONSIDERATIONS

- Available as nasal solutions, nebulizer solution, PO
- Available as generic only
- Full therapeutic effect may take several weeks
- PO: take 30 min ac, do not crush
- Not appropriate for acute asthma
- Rx

• •

ADVERSE EFFECTS

In the absence of
alcohol:
- Drowsiness
- Headache
- Restlessness

In the presence of
alcohol:
- Flushing
- Chest pain
- Heart dysrhythmias

- Hypotension
- Seizures
- Throbbing in head and neck
- Sweating

NURSING CONSIDERATIONS

- Causes severe hypersensitivity
- Onset may be delayed up to 12 hr; single dose may be effective for 1–2 weeks
- Avoid alcohol in any form: in foods, sauces, or other meds, such as cough syrups or tonics
- Avoid vinegar, paregoric, skin products, liniments, or lotions containing alcohol
- Do not begin treatment for at least 12 hr after drinking alcohol
- Rx

DARBEPOETIN ALFA
(dar-buh-<u>poe</u>-uh-tin <u>al</u>-fuh)

Purpose: treatment of anemia caused by disease

• •

EPOETIN ALFA
(i-<u>poe</u>-uh-tin <u>al</u>-fuh)

Purpose: treatment of anemia caused by disease

ADVERSE EFFECTS

Headache, fatigue	Mucositis, stomatitis	Alopecia
Chest pain	Myalgias	Rash, urticaria
Hypertension	Fever	Seizures
Nausea, vomiting, diarrhea	Dyspnea, cough	Stinging at injection site
	Sore throat	

NURSING CONSIDERATIONS

- Given IM
- Contraindicated in uncontrolled hypertension
- Do not use in breast, non-small-cell lung, head and neck, lymphoid, cervical cancers
- Use with caution in cardiac disease, seizures, porphyria
- May increase risk of death
- Monitor BP and hemoglobin
- Teach client to give injections
- Rx

• •

ADVERSE EFFECTS

Headache, fatigue	Pruritus
Coldness, sweating	Bone pain
Hypertension	Cough
Hypertensive encephalopathy	Seizures
Change in heart rate	Thrombosis

NURSING CONSIDERATIONS

- Therapeutic response in 2–4 weeks
- SubQ: do not shake vial
- IV: do not dilute or administer with other solutions
- Use with caution in kidney disease
- Increased risk of tumor growth with some cancers
- Avoid driving and hazardous activities until reaction known
- Rx

MINOXIDIL (TOPICAL)
(mi-<u>nox</u>-i-dill)

Purpose: treatment of alopecia

• •

CARBONYL IRON
(<u>kar</u>-buh-nill)

Purpose: treatment of iron deficiency anemia, prophylaxis for iron deficiency in pregnancy

ADVERSE EFFECTS

Edema   Rash
Increase in body hair   Headache, fatigue

NURSING CONSIDERATIONS

- Do not use on children or infants
- Avoid contact with eyes, mucous membranes, sensitive skin areas
- Increasing dosage does not speed growth
- Treatment must continue for long-term
- OTC, Rx

• •

ADVERSE EFFECTS

Nausea, constipation   Black or discolored stools
Epigastric pain

NURSING CONSIDERATIONS

- Contains 100% elemental iron
- Liquid preparation may stain teeth
- Keep client upright for 15–30 min to avoid esophageal corrosion; take 1 hr before bedtime
- Iron overdose is a leading cause of poisoning in children
- Stools will become black or dark green
- Notify provider if stools are tarry or blood-streaked; indicates GI bleeding
- Do not substitute one iron salt for another because iron content differs
- Do not take within 1 hr before or 2 hr after antacids, eggs, whole-grain bread or cereal, milk, coffee, or tea
- OTC, Rx

FERRIC GLUCONATE COMPLEX
(<u>fair</u>-ik <u>gloo</u>-kuh-nate)

Purpose: treatment of iron deficiency anemia in dialysis clients

· ·

FERROUS SULFATE
(<u>fair</u>-us <u>sull</u>-fate)

Purpose: treatment of iron deficiency

ADVERSE EFFECTS

Hypotension
Flushing

NURSING CONSIDERATIONS

- Given IV
- Notify provider if difficulty breathing or oral edema occurs
- Notify provider if stools are tarry or blood-streaked; indicates GI bleeding
- Do not mix with other meds; may be mixed only with normal saline solution
- Iron overdose is a leading cause of poisoning in children
- Rx

• •

ADVERSE EFFECTS

GI upset	Serious toxicity with high doses
Constipation	Liver damage with high doses

NURSING CONSIDERATIONS

- Liquid preparation may stain teeth
- Administer between meals if possible
- Give with food to reduce GI effects; reduces absorption
- Antacid use may reduce absorption
- Give with vitamin C to improve absorption
- May cause black stools
- Lower daily doses in older adult clients to decrease GI upset
- Iron overdose is a leading cause of poisoning in children
- May be given prophylactically during pregnancy to reduce anemia
- OTC, Rx

POTASSIUM CHLORIDE
(puh-<u>tass</u>-ee-um <u>klor</u>-ide)

Purpose: prevention and treatment of hypokalemia

• •

NALOXONE HCL
(na-<u>lox</u>-own)

Purpose: treatment of respiratory depression induced by opiates

ADVERSE EFFECTS

Nausea, vomiting
Confusion
Cramps, diarrhea

Cardiac dysrhythmias
Oliguria

NURSING CONSIDERATIONS

- PO: onset 30 min; remain upright for 30 min after administration
- IV: onset immediate
- Do not infuse faster than 10 mg/hr in adults
- Do not give IM, subQ, IV push
- Dilute liquid prior to giving via NG
- Monitor IV infusions for extravasation: may sting or burn
- Report hyperkalemia: lethargy, confusion, GI symptoms, fainting, decreased urinary output
- Avoid OTC antacids, salt substitutes, analgesics, vitamins unless directed by provider
- OTC, Rx

• •

ADVERSE EFFECTS

Nervousness
Tremor
Rapid pulse

Nausea, vomiting
Dyspnea

NURSING CONSIDERATIONS

- IM and subQ onset in 2–5 min; IV 1–2 min
- Have emergency support equipment available
- Monitor for bleeding in surgical and obstetric clients
- Withdrawal symptoms in narcotic-dependent clients: restlessness, muscle spasms, tearing
- OTC, Rx

NALTREXONE
(nal-<u>trex</u>-own)

Purpose: opioid cessation, treatment of opioid-use and alcohol-use disorders

• •

CHOLECALCIFEROL (AQUEOUS VITAMIN D₃)
(koe-luh-kal-<u>sif</u>-uh-rall)

Purpose: treatment of vitamin D deficiency in rickets, osteomalacia, osteoporosis, and hypoparathyroidism

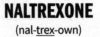

ADVERSE EFFECTS

Insomnia, somnolence

Anxiety, nervousness, irritability

Headache, fatigue

Dizziness, syncope

Depression

Suicidal ideation

GI disturbance

Anorexia, dry mouth

Constipation

Delayed ejaculation, decreased potency

Muscle, joint, and back pain

Muscle cramps

Rash, injection-site reaction

Chills, flulike symptoms

NURSING CONSIDERATIONS

- Given IM or PO
- Contraindicated in opioid dependency
- Client must be opioid-free before taking med
- Discontinue if acute hepatitis develops
- Monitor for depression, suicidal ideation
- Monitor respirations initially; may cause respiratory depression
- Rx

• •

ADVERSE EFFECTS

Hypercalcemia   Nephrotoxicity   Hypervitaminosis D
Nephrolithiasis   Hyperphosphatemia

NURSING CONSIDERATIONS

- Do not crush or chew
- Monitor levels of alkaline phosphatase, BUN, free and total calcium, magnesium, phosphate
- Obese clients may require higher doses for effectiveness
- Dark-skinned clients may require higher doses
- Rx, OTC

CYANOCOBALAMIN
(<u>sye</u>-an-oh-koe-<u>bal</u>-a-min)

Purpose: treatment of vitamin B$_{12}$ deficiency, pernicious anemia, hemorrhage, kidney disease, and liver disease

• •

ERGOCALCIFEROL
(<u>er</u>-goe-kal-<u>sif</u>-uh-role)

Purpose: treatment of vitamin D deficiency, rickets, osteomalacia, osteoporosis, and hypoparathyroidism

ADVERSE EFFECTS

Diarrhea
Hypokalemia

Pulmonary edema
Itching

NURSING CONSIDERATIONS

- IM, subQ, nasal: peak 3–10 days
- May take with fruit juice to disguise taste
- Meats, seafood, egg yolk, fermented cheeses are good dietary sources of vitamin B_{12}
- OTC, Rx

. . . .

ADVERSE EFFECTS

Metallic taste, dry mouth
Hypervitaminosis D
Headache
Fatigue, weakness

Nephrotoxicity
Hypertension
Photophobia

NURSING CONSIDERATIONS

- If dose missed, omit
- Avoid use of antacids and laxatives containing magnesium
- Mineral oil interferes with absorption
- Rx, OTC

FOLIC ACID
(<u>foe</u>-lik)

Purpose: treatment of anemia, liver disease, alcoholism, hemolysis, and intestinal obstruction; reduction of embryonic neural tube defects

· ·

HYDROXOCOBALAMIN
(hye-<u>drox</u>-o-ko-<u>bal</u>-a-min)

Purpose: treatment of vitamin B_{12} deficiency, pernicious anemia, malabsorption syndrome, hemolytic anemia, kidney disease, liver disease, and cyanide poisoning

ADVERSE EFFECTS

Bronchospasm

Conduction, irritability

Anorexia

Bitter taste

Pruritus

NURSING CONSIDERATIONS

- Important to prevent fetal neural tube defects
- Bran, yeast, dried beans, nuts, fruits, fresh vegetables, asparagus are good dietary sources of iron
- May cause urine to turn bright yellow
- OTC

• •

ADVERSE EFFECTS

Diarrhea

Flushing

Pulmonary edema

Hypokalemia

Itching at injection site

NURSING CONSIDERATIONS

- IM, subQ: peak 3–10 days
- Meats, seafood, egg yolk, fermented cheeses are good dietary sources of vitamin B_{12}
- OTC, Rx

DTAP/TDAP/TD VACCINE
(<u>dee</u>-tap/<u>tee</u>-dap/tee-dee)

Purpose: prevention of diphtheria, tetanus, and acellular pertussis
(whooping cough)

• •

HAEMOPHILUS INFLUENZAE
TYPE B (HIB) VACCINE
(hee-<u>mah</u>-fill-us in-floo-<u>en</u>-zee)

Purpose: prevention of Haemophilus influenzae type B infection

ADVERSE EFFECTS

Fever

Redness, swelling, or soreness
at injection site

Fussiness

Serious allergic reaction in less
than 1 per 1 million doses

NURSING CONSIDERATIONS

- Contains only portions of the bacteria; cannot cause infection
- DTaP for children less than 7 years
- Tdap for older children and adults
- Td contains no pertussis; for older children and adults
- Control fever with aspirin-free pain reliever, esp. in child with
  seizures
- Children: administer in 5 doses
- Rx

• •

ADVERSE EFFECTS

Injection-site redness, warmth (uncommon)

Dizziness, shoulder pain (very rare)

NURSING CONSIDERATIONS

- Contains only portions of the bacteria; cannot cause infection
- Children: administer in 3 or 4 doses (depends on brand)
- Rx

HEPATITIS A VACCINE

(hep-uh-<u>tye</u>-tis)

Purpose: prevention of hepatitis A infection

. . . .

HEPATITIS B VACCINE

(hep-uh-<u>tye</u>-tis)

Purpose: prevention of hepatitis B infection

ADVERSE EFFECTS

Soreness at injection site (50% in adults, 17% in children)
Headache (17% in adults, 4% in children)
Serious allergic reaction rare

NURSING CONSIDERATIONS

- Contains the whole, but killed virus; cannot cause infection
- Two doses needed for lasting protection
- Rx

• •

ADVERSE EFFECTS

Soreness at injection site (25%)
Severe allergic reaction in 1 per 1.1 million doses

NURSING CONSIDERATIONS

- Contains only portions of virus; cannot cause infection
- Infants: administer in 3 doses
- Rx

HUMAN PAPILLOMAVIRUS (HPV) VACCINE
(<u>hyoo</u>-man pap-ill-<u>oh</u>-mah-<u>vye</u>-rus)

*Purpose: prevention of infection with HPV types 6, 11, 16, and 18, which
cause cervical cancer*

• •

INFLUENZA VACCINE
(in-floo-<u>en</u>-zuh)

Purpose: prevention of seasonal flu infection

ADVERSE EFFECTS

Pain at injection site
Redness or swelling
Headache or fatigue

GI symptoms
Muscle or joint pain

NURSING CONSIDERATIONS

- Contains only portions of the virus; cannot cause infection
- Recommended for children age 11–12
- Given as 3-dose series
- Rx

ADVERSE EFFECTS

Injection-site swelling, soreness
Flulike symptoms (nasal spray)

NURSING CONSIDERATIONS

- IM: injection contains the whole but killed virus; cannot cause infection
- Nasal spray: contains live, weakened viruses; designed to trigger a mild infection, inducing immunity
- Serious allergic reaction in less than 1 per 1 million doses
- OTC

MEASLES, MUMPS, & RUBELLA (MMR) VACCINE
(<u>mee</u>-zulls mumps and roo-<u>bell</u>-uh)

Purpose: prevention of infection with measles, mumps, and rubella ("German measles")

● ●

MENINGOCOCCAL VACCINE
(men-<u>ing</u>-guh-<u>cok</u>-ull)

Purpose: prevention of meningitis infection

ADVERSE EFFECTS

Fever

NURSING CONSIDERATIONS

- Contains live but weakened viruses; can cause the actual diseases
- Serious allergic reactions in less than 1 in 1 million doses
- Children: administer in 2 doses
- Rx

. . . .

ADVERSE EFFECTS

Redness or pain at injection site

NURSING CONSIDERATIONS

- Contains only portions of the bacteria; cannot cause infection
- Adolescents: 2 doses recommended
- Serious allergic reactions very rare
- Rx

PNEUMOCOCCAL CONJUGATE VACCINE (PCV13)
(<u>new</u>-moe-cok-ull <u>con</u>-juh-get)

Purpose: prevention of infections caused by Streptococcus pneumoniae

• •

PNEUMOCOCCAL POLYSACCHARIDE VACCINE (PPSV23)
(<u>new</u>-moe-cok-ull pol-ee-<u>sak</u>-uh-ride)

Purpose: prevention of infections caused by Streptococcus pneumoniae

ADVERSE EFFECTS

Children: drowsiness, anorexia, injection-site redness or tenderness
Children: irritability

Children: mild fever, swelling at injection site
Adults: mild reactions

NURSING CONSIDERATIONS

- Contains only portions of the bacteria; cannot cause disease
- For children under age 2
- For adults age 50 and older
- Protects against 13 strains of pneumococcal bacteria
- Rx

• •

ADVERSE EFFECTS

Children: drowsiness, anorexia, injection-site redness or tenderness
Children: irritability

Children: mild fever, swelling at injection site
Adults: mild reactions

NURSING CONSIDERATIONS

- Contains only portions of the bacteria; cannot cause disease
- For at-risk children over age 2 years
- For adults age 50 and older
- Protects against 23 strains of pneumococcal bacteria
- Rx

POLIO VACCINE
(<u>poe</u>-lee-oh)

Purpose: prevention of polio infection

. . . .

ROTAVIRUS VACCINE
(<u>row</u>-tuh-vye-rus)

Purpose: prevention of rotavirus infection

ADVERSE EFFECTS

Mild fever
Soreness at injection site
Minimal risk of allergic reaction

NURSING CONSIDERATIONS

- Contains whole but killed virus; cannot cause disease
- Children: administer in 4 doses
- Rx

• •

ADVERSE EFFECTS

Irritability
GI upset

NURSING CONSIDERATIONS

- Contains the whole live virus; designed to trigger low-grade infection to create immunity
- Administer PO: oral liquid vaccine
- Infants: administer in 2 or 3 doses (depends on brand)
- Rx

VARICELLA VACCINE
(<u>vair</u>-i-sell-ah)

Purpose: prevention of varicella-zoster (chickenpox) infection

· ·

Vasoactive Medications
Vasodilators/Antihypertensives, Intravenous

NICARDIPINE
(nye-<u>kar</u>-di-peen)

Purpose: treatment of angina and hypertension

ADVERSE EFFECTS

Soreness at injection site
Fever
Rash (rare)

NURSING CONSIDERATIONS

- Contains live but weakened virus; immunization can cause a mild case of the disease
- Counsel client to avoid contact with newborns, pregnant women, and immunocompromised individuals immediately after injection
- Rx

• •

ADVERSE EFFECTS

Tachycardia, hypotension
Heart block
Edema
Flushing
Rash

Confusion, headache, dizziness
Insomnia, nervousness
Fatigue

Constipation
Diarrhea, dyspepsia
Elevated liver enzymes

NURSING CONSIDERATIONS

- Contraindicated in severe hypotension or heart block greater than first degree
- Use with caution in liver or kidney impairment, bradycardia, heart failure, cardiogenic shock
- Monitor BP for sudden decrease
- Do not use in pregnancy; use with caution in breastfeeding
- Do not stop abruptly; taper over a few weeks
- Avoid grapefruit products, high-fat foods
- Rx

NITROPRUSSIDE
(nye-troe-<u>pruss</u>-ide)

Purpose: treatment of hypertensive emergency, controlled hypotension for surgery and acute heart failure

· ·

DOBUTAMINE
(doe-<u>byoo</u>-ta-meen)

Purpose: management of heart failure and supraventricular arrhythmias, including supraventricular tachycardia and atrial fibrillation

ADVERSE EFFECTS

Headache, dizziness

Increased ICP, loss of
consciousness

Apprehension, restlessness

Bradycardia, tachycardia,
palpitations, ECG changes

GI disturbance

Decreased platelet aggregation

Metabolic acidosis

Hypothyroidism

Muscle twitching

Diaphoresis, flushing, rash

Thiocyanate toxicity

Cyanide toxicity

NURSING CONSIDERATIONS

* IV: give diluted in 250–1,000 mL fluid; monitor BP continuously
* Keep in supine position when starting or titrating therapy
* May cause severe hypotension
* Monitor for venous streaking, irritation at IV site
* Adjust dose for clients taking other antihypertensives
* Do not use in pregnancy or breastfeeding
* Many medication interactions
* Protect med from light
* Rx

• •

ADVERSE EFFECTS

Dysrhythmias

Chest pain

Nausea, vomiting, diarrhea

Headache

Fever

Mental disturbances

Visual changes

NURSING CONSIDERATIONS

* IV: give in a dilution
* Available as generic only
* Increases AV node conduction
* May cause severe hypotension
* Monitor with continuous ECG and BP
* Do not use in pregnancy or breastfeeding unless clearly needed
* Rx

DOPAMINE
(<u>doe</u>-pa-meen)

Purpose: correction of hemodynamic imbalances in shock, trauma, septicemia, cardiac surgical procedures, spinal anesthesia, medication reactions, kidney failure, and heart failure

• •

EPINEPHRINE
(ep-i-<u>nef</u>-rin)

Purpose: emergency treatment of anaphylaxis; treatment of shock, trauma, and septicemia; prophylaxis for cardiac surgical procedures and spinal anesthesia; management of medication reactions, kidney failure, and heart failure

ADVERSE EFFECTS

Ventricular dysrhythmias
Tachycardia, bradycardia
Angina, palpitations
Widened QRS complex
Hyper/hypotension,
vasoconstriction
Anxiety, headache

Dyspnea, nausea
Azotemia
Phlebitis
Peripheral cyanosis, gangrene of
extremities
Dysuria with ephedrine
Decreased urine output

NURSING CONSIDERATIONS

- Available as generic only
- Administer in large vein; monitor to prevent extravasation
- Contraindicated in hypersensitivity, pheochromocytoma, uncorrected tachydysrhythmias, ventricular fibrillation
- Use with extreme caution within 2–3 weeks of MAOI
- Use with caution in hyperthyroidism, bradycardia, partial heart block, myocardial disease, severe arteriosclerosis
- Use with caution in pregnancy, breastfeeding, sulfite allergy
- Rx

• •

ADVERSE EFFECTS

Ventricular dysrhythmias
Tachycardia, bradycardia
Angina, palpitations
Conduction abnormalities
Widened QRS complex
Hyper/hypotension,
vasoconstriction

Anxiety, headache
Dyspnea, nausea
Azotemia, dysuria
Phlebitis, thrombocytopenia
Peripheral cyanosis, gangrene
of extremities
Hypokalemia

NURSING CONSIDERATIONS

- Administer in large vein; carefully monitor BP
- Contraindicated in hypersensitivity, pheochromocytoma, uncorrected tachydysrhythmias, ventricular fibrillation
- Use with extreme caution within 2–3 weeks of MAOI
- Use with caution in hyperthyroidism, bradycardia, partial heart block, myocardial disease, severe arteriosclerosis
- Use with caution in pregnancy, breastfeeding, sulfite allergy
- Teach use if using autoinjector
- Rx

NOREPINEPHRINE

(nor-ep-i-<u>nef</u>-rin)

Purpose: treatment of shock, trauma, and septicemia; prophylaxis for cardiac surgical procedures and spinal anesthesia; management of medication reactions, kidney failure, and heart failure

● ●

VASOPRESSIN (ANTIDIURETIC HORMONE [ADH])

(vay-zo-<u>press</u>-in)

Purpose: vasoconstriction

ADVERSE EFFECTS

Ventricular dysrhythmias

Tachycardia, bradycardia

Angina, palpitations

Conduction abnormalities

Widened QRS complex

Hyper/hypotension, vasoconstriction

Anxiety, headache

Dyspnea, nausea

Azotemia, dysuria

Phlebitis, thrombocytopenia

Peripheral cyanosis, gangrene of extremities

Hypokalemia

NURSING CONSIDERATIONS

- IV: into large vein to avoid extravasation; decrease gradually
- Contraindicated in pheochromocytoma, uncorrected tachydysrhythmias, ventricular fibrillation
- Use with extreme caution within 2–3 weeks of MAOI
- Use with caution in hyperthyroidism, bradycardia, partial heart block, myocardial disease, severe arteriosclerosis
- Use with caution in pregnancy, breastfeeding, sulfite allergy
- Not the same as epinephrine; use atropine to reverse effects
- Rx

• •

ADVERSE EFFECTS

Headache, vertigo

Hemorrhagic shock

Heart failure, atrial fibrillation, bradycardia

Myocardial ischemia

Decreased cardiac output

Distal limb ischemia

Thrombocytopenia

Mesenteric ischemia

Acute kidney injury

Hyponatremia

Cutaneous gangrene

Water intoxication

NURSING CONSIDERATIONS

- Give IM or subQ
- Extravasation may result in severe tissue damage
- Use with caution in older adult, pediatric, pregnant, breastfeeding clients
- Monitor for hypersensitivity reactions, bleeding, palpitations, signs/symptoms of ischemia
- Monitor urine specific gravity, I&O
- Monitor ECG and fluid/electrolyte status periodically
- Rx

DROSPIRENONE/ETHINYL ESTRADIOL
(drah-<u>speer</u>-uh-noan/eh-<u>thye</u>-nul es-truh-<u>dye</u>-ol)

Purpose: contraception, treatment of acne

• •

ETHINYL ESTRADIOL/ETHYNODIOL
(eh-<u>thye</u>-nul es-truh-<u>dye</u>-ol/eth-i-noe-<u>dye</u>-ol)

Purpose: contraception, treatment of acne

ADVERSE EFFECTS

Headache

Vaginal itching, discharge, or
  yeast infection

Nausea

Breakthrough bleeding

Increase in BP

Weight gain

Symptoms of depression

NURSING CONSIDERATIONS

- Monophasic oral contraceptive
- Take at the same time daily, once a day
- Avoid smoking (increases risk of adverse cardiovascular events)
- Counsel client that this med does not protect against STIs or HIV
- Teach client to promptly report any visual disturbances, unusual bleeding, chest or leg pain, change in coordination, dyspnea, or severe headache
- May increase risk of cardiovascular events including MI and stroke
- St. John's wort and antibiotics may decrease effectiveness
- Rx

• •

ADVERSE EFFECTS

Headache

Breakthrough bleeding,
  spotting

Dizziness

Nausea

Contact lens intolerance

NURSING CONSIDERATIONS

- Monophasic oral contraceptive
- Take at same time each day
- Counsel client that this med does not protect against STIs or HIV
- Contact provider if unusual bleeding, severe headache, difficulty breathing, changes in vision/coordination, chest/leg pain
- Avoid smoking (increases risk of adverse cardiovascular events)
- Stop med for at least 1 week before surgery to decrease risk of thromboembolism
- St. John's wort and antibiotics may decrease effectiveness
- Rx

ETHINYL ESTRADIOL/NORETHINDRONE
(eh-<u>thye</u>-nul es-truh-<u>dye</u>-ol/nor-<u>eth</u>-in-drone)

Purpose: contraception, treatment of acne

• •

NORETHINDRONE
(nor-<u>eth</u>-in-drone)

Purpose: contraception, treatment of abnormal bleeding and endometriosis

ADVERSE EFFECTS

Nausea
Headache
Breakthrough bleeding

Contact lens intolerance
Dizziness

NURSING CONSIDERATIONS

- Triphasic oral contraceptive
- St. John's wort and antibiotics may decrease effectiveness
- Counsel client that med does not protect against STIs or HIV
- Take at same time each day
- Contact provider if breast lumps, vaginal bleeding, edema, jaundice, dark urine, clay-colored stools, dyspnea, headache, blurred vision, abdominal pain, numbness or stiffness in legs, chest pain, tenderness with redness and swelling in extremities
- Contact provider if weekly weight gain is over 5 pounds
- Avoid smoking (increases risk of adverse cardiovascular events)
- Can take with food or milk to decrease GI upset
- Rx

• •

ADVERSE EFFECTS

Nausea
Headache

Dizziness
Breakthrough bleeding

NURSING CONSIDERATIONS

- Progestin oral contraceptive
- Counsel client that this med does not protect against STIs or HIV
- Contact provider if breast lumps, vaginal bleeding, edema, jaundice, dark urine, clay-colored stools, dyspnea, headache, blurred vision, abdominal pain, numbness or stiffness in legs, chest pain, tenderness with redness and swelling in extremities
- Contact provider if weekly weight gain is over 5 pounds
- Can take with food or milk to decrease GI upset
- Avoid smoking, which increases risk of serious cardiovascular events
- Rx

CONJUGATED ESTROGENS
(<u>kon</u>-juh-gate-id <u>ess</u>-truh-jenz)

Purpose: treatment of menopausal symptoms and atrophic vaginitis, palliative therapy for breast cancer and prostatic cancer

• •

ESTRADIOL (ORAL), ESTRADIOL VALERATE
(es-truh-<u>dye</u>-ol, es-truh-<u>dye</u>-ol <u>val</u>-uh-rate)

Purpose: treatment of menopausal symptoms, inoperable breast cancer, prostatic cancer, and atrophic vaginitis; prevention of osteoporosis

ADVERSE EFFECTS

Nausea	Gynecomastia	Impotence
Contact lens intolerance	Testicular atrophy	Dementia

NURSING CONSIDERATIONS

- IM: inject deep into large muscle mass
- PO: can take with food or milk to decrease GI upset
- May increase risk of cardiovascular events
- May increase risk of endometrial cancer and ovarian cancer
- Contact provider if breast lumps, vaginal bleeding, edema, jaundice, dark urine, clay-colored stools, dyspnea, headache, blurred vision, abdominal pain, numbness or stiffness in legs, chest pain, tenderness with redness and swelling in extremities
- Men should contact provider to report impotence or gynecomastia
- Contact provider if weekly weight gain is over 5 pounds
- Rx

• •

ADVERSE EFFECTS

Nausea	Weight gain	MI, hypertension
Gynecomastia	Testicular atrophy	Thromboembolism
Contact lens intolerance	Impotence	Hypercalcemia
	Headache, dizziness	Hyperglycemia

NURSING CONSIDERATIONS

- IM: inject deep into large muscle mass
- Contact provider if breast lumps, vaginal bleeding, edema, jaundice, dark urine, clay-colored stools, dyspnea, headache, blurred vision, abdominal pain, numbness or stiffness in legs, chest pain, tenderness with redness and swelling in extremities
- Men should contact provider to report impotence or gynecomastia
- Contact provider if weekly weight gain is over 5 pounds
- Can take with food or milk to decrease GI upset
- May increase risk of endometrial cancer, breast cancer, adverse cardiovascular events
- Rx

CLOMIPHENE CITRATE
(<u>klo</u>-muh-feen <u>sih</u>-trate)

Purpose: stimulation of ovulation to increase fertility

• •

MEDROXYPROGESTERONE ACETATE
(meh-<u>drox</u>-ee-proe-<u>jess</u>-tuh-rone <u>ass</u>-uh-tate)

Purpose: contraception; management of uterine bleeding, secondary amenorrhea, endometrial cancer, and kidney cancer

ADVERSE EFFECTS

Vasomotor flushes
Breast discomfort
Heavy menses
Depression
Headache
Nausea, vomiting
Constipation, bloating

Spontaneous abortion
Multiple ovulations
Enlarged ovaries with multiple
  follicular cysts
Ophthalmic "floaters," diplopia
Deep vein thrombosis
Hepatitis

NURSING CONSIDERATIONS

- May be available as generic only
- Teach client to immediately report abnormal bleeding, pelvic pain, hot flashes
- Client should stop med if pregnancy is suspected
- Rx

• •

ADVERSE EFFECTS

Nausea
Diplopia
Testicular atrophy
Dizziness
Impotence

GI upset
Galactorrhea
Depression
Hyperglycemia
Stroke/MI

Photosensitivity
Decreased bone
  density
Dementia

NURSING CONSIDERATIONS

- IM: inject deep into large muscle mass; rotate sites, injection may be painful
- May increase risk of ovarian cancer, breast cancer, adverse cardiovascular events
- Counsel client that this med does not protect against STIs or HIV
- Contact provider if weekly weight gain is over 5 pounds
- Contact provider if swelling in calves, sudden chest pain, or SOB
- Rx

APPENDIX A:
Controlled Substance Schedules

Medications regulated by the Controlled Substances Act of 1970 are given these classifications.

Schedule I: High abuse potential and no accepted medical use. Examples include heroin, marijuana, peyote, Ecstasy, and LSD.

Schedule II: High abuse potential with severe dependence liability. Examples include narcotics, amphetamines, and some barbiturates.

Schedule III: Less abuse potential than Schedule II medications and moderate dependence liability. Examples include nonbarbiturate sedatives, nonamphetamine stimulants, anabolic steroids, and limited amounts of certain narcotics.

Schedule IV: Less abuse potential than Schedule III medications and limited dependence liability. Examples include some sedatives, anxiolytics, and nonnarcotic analgesics.

Schedule V: Limited abuse potential. Examples include small amounts of narcotics, such as codeine, used as antidiarrheals or antitussives.

APPENDIX B:

Special Considerations

Black box warning, also known as boxed warning: Food and Drug Administration (FDA) warning placed by the manufacturer on a prescription medication package insert. It communicates that the medication carries a significant risk of serious or even life-threatening adverse effects.

Off-label use: Use of medications for an unapproved indication or in an unapproved age group, unapproved dosage, or unapproved route of administration.

Pregnancy and lactation: Prior to June 2015, the FDA required that most prescribed medications be labeled for risk according to letter categories A (remote possibility of fetal harm), B, C, D, and X (studies show evidence of fetal risk). In June 2015, the FDA changed to a system in which providers assess the benefit versus the risk of a given medication for individual pregnant women and nursing mothers. FDA guidelines call for subsequent counseling of pregnant and lactating clients, "allowing them to make informed and educated decisions for themselves and their children." The FDA created a pregnancy exposure registry to collect and maintain data on the effects of approved medications prescribed to and used by pregnant women (FDA *Pregnancy and Lactation Labeling Final Rule*, December 3, 2014).

APPENDIX C:

Common Medical Abbreviations

ABC—airway, breathing, circulation

abd.—abdomen

ABG—arterial blood gas

ABO—system of classifying blood groups

ac—before meals

ACE—angiotensin-converting enzyme

ACS—acute compartment syndrome

ACTH—adrenocorticotropic hormone

ADH—antidiuretic hormone

ADHD—attention deficit hyperactivity disorder

ADL—activities of daily living

ad lib—freely, as desired

AFP—alpha-fetoprotein

AIDS—acquired immunodeficiency syndrome

AKA—above-the-knee amputation

ALL—acute lymphocytic leukemia

ALS—amyotrophic lateral sclerosis

ALT—alanine transaminase (formerly SGPT)

AMI—antibody-mediated immunity

AML—acute myelogenous leukemia

amt.—amount

ANA—antinuclear antibody

ANS—autonomic nervous system

AP—anteroposterior

A&P—anterior and posterior

APC—atrial premature contraction

aq.—water

ARDS—adult respiratory distress syndrome

ASD—atrial septal defect

ASHD—atherosclerotic heart disease

AST—aspartate aminotransferase (formerly SGOT)

ATP—adenosine triphosphate

AV—atrioventricular

BCG—bacille Calmette-Guérin

bid—two times a day

BKA—below-the-knee amputation

BLS—basic life support

BMR—basal metabolic rate

BP—blood pressure

BPH—benign prostatic hyperplasia

bpm—beats per minute

BPR—bathroom privileges

BSA—body surface area

BUN—blood urea nitrogen

C—centigrade, Celsius

c—with

Ca—calcium

CA—cancer

CABG—coronary artery bypass graft

CAD—coronary artery disease

CAPD—continuous ambulatory peritoneal dialysis

caps—capsules

CBC—complete blood count

CC—chief complaint

CCU—coronary care unit, critical care unit

CDC—Centers for Disease Control and Prevention

CK—creatine kinase

Cl—chloride

CLL—chronic lymphocytic leukemia

cm—centimeter

CMV—cytomegalovirus infection

CNS—central nervous system

CO—carbon monoxide, cardiac output

CO$_2$—carbon dioxide

comp—compound

cont—continuous

COPD—chronic obstructive pulmonary disease

CP—cerebral palsy

CPAP—continuous positive airway pressure

CPK—creatine phosphokinase

CPR—cardiopulmonary resuscitation

CRP—C-reactive protein

C&S—culture and sensitivity

CSF—cerebrospinal fluid

CT—computed tomography

CTD—connective tissue disease

CTS—carpal tunnel syndrome

cu—cubic

CVA—cerebrovascular accident, costovertebral angle

CVC—central venous catheter

CVP—central venous pressure

D&C—dilation and curettage

DIC—disseminated intravascular coagulation

DIFF—differential blood count

dil.—dilute

DJD—degenerative joint disease

DKA—diabetic ketoacidosis

dL—deciliter (100 mL)

DM—diabetes mellitus

DNA—deoxyribonucleic acid

DNR—do not resuscitate

DO—doctor of osteopathy

DOE—dyspnea on exertion

DPT—vaccine for diphtheria, pertussis, tetanus

DVT—deep vein thrombosis

D/W—dextrose in water

Dx—diagnosis

ECF—extracellular fluid

ECG, EKG—electrocardiogram

ECT—electroconvulsive therapy

ED—emergency department

EEG—electroencephalogram

EMD—electromechanical dissociation

EMG—electromyography

ENT—ear, nose, and throat

EPS—extrapyramidal symptoms

ESR—erythrocyte sedimentation rate

ESRD—end-stage renal disease

ET—endotracheal tube

F—Fahrenheit

FBD—fibrocystic breast disease

FBS—fasting blood sugar

FDA—U.S. Food and Drug Administration

FFP—fresh frozen plasma

fl—fluid

4 × 4—piece of gauze 4 inches long by 4 inches wide used for dressings

FSH—follicle-stimulating hormone

ft.—foot, feet (unit of measure)

FUO—fever of undetermined origin

g—gram

GB—gallbladder

GFR—glomerular filtration rate

GH—growth hormone

GI—gastrointestinal

gr—grain

GSC—Glasgow coma scale

GTT—glucose tolerance test

gtts—drops

GU—genitourinary

GYN—gynecological

h, hr—hour or hours

(H)—hypodermically

Hb or Hgb—hemoglobin

hCG—human chorionic gonadotropin

HCO₃—bicarbonate

HCO_3^-—bicarbonate

Hct—hematocrit

HD—hemodialysis

HDL—high-density lipoproteins

HF—heart failure

Hg—mercury

Hgb—hemoglobin

HGH—human growth hormone

HHNC—hyperglycemia hyperosmolar nonketotic coma

HIV—human immunodeficiency virus

HLA—human leukocyte antigen

HR—heart rate

HSV—herpes simplex virus

HTN—hypertension

H₂O—water

Hx—history

Hz—hertz (cycles/second)

IABP—intra-aortic balloon pump

IBS—irritable bowel syndrome

ICF—intracellular fluid

ICP—intracranial pressure

ICS—intercostal space

ICU—intensive care unit

IDDM—insulin-dependent diabetes mellitus

IgA—immunoglobulin A

IM—intramuscular

I&O—intake and output

IOP—intraocular pressure

IPG—impedance plethysmogram

IPPB—intermittent positive-pressure breathing

IUD—intrauterine device

IV—intravenous

IVC—intraventricular catheter

IVP—intravenous pyelogram

JRA—juvenile rheumatoid arthritis

K⁺—potassium

kcal—kilocalorie (food calorie)

kg—kilogram

KO, KVO—keep vein open

KS—Kaposi sarcoma

KUB—kidneys, ureters, bladder

L, l—liter

lab—laboratory

lb—pound

LBBB—left bundle branch block

LDH—lactate dehydrogenase

LDL—low-density lipoproteins

LE—lupus erythematosus

LH—luteinizing hormone

liq—liquid

LLQ—left lower quadrant

LOC—level of consciousness

LP—lumbar puncture

LPN, LVN—licensed practical nurse, licensed vocational nurse

LTC—long-term care

LUQ—left upper quadrant

LV—left ventricle

m—meter, micron

MAOI—monoamine oxidase inhibitor

MAST—military antishock trousers

mcg—microgram

MCH—mean corpuscular hemoglobin

MCV—mean corpuscular volume

MD—muscular dystrophy, medical doctor

MDI—metered-dose inhaler

mEq—milliequivalent

mg—milligram

Mg—magnesium

MG—myasthenia gravis

MI—myocardial infarction

mL—milliliter

mm—millimeter

MMR—vaccine for measles, mumps, and rubella

MRI—magnetic resonance imaging

MS—multiple sclerosis

N—nitrogen, normal (strength of solution)

NIDDM—non-insulin-dependent diabetes mellitus

Na$^+$—sodium

NaCl—sodium chloride

NANDA—North American Nursing Diagnosis Association

NG—nasogastric

NGT—nasogastric tube

NLN—National League for Nursing

noc—at night

NPO—nothing by mouth

NS—normal saline

NSR—normal sinus rhythm (cardiac)

NSAIDs—nonsteroidal anti-inflammatory drugs

NSNA—National Student Nurses' Association

NST—nonstress test

O₂—oxygen

OB-GYN—obstetrics and gynecology

OCT—oxytocin challenge test

OOB—out of bed

OPC—outpatient clinic

OR—operating room

os—by mouth

OSHA—Occupational Safety and Health Administration

OTC—over-the-counter (medication obtained without prescription)

oz—ounce

p—with

P—pulse, pressure, phosphorus

PA chest—posterior-anterior chest x-ray

PAC—premature atrial complexes

PaCO₂—partial pressure of carbon dioxide in arterial blood

PaO₂—partial pressure of oxygen in arterial blood

PAD—peripheral artery disease

Pap—Papanicolaou smear

PBI—protein-bound iodine

pc—after meals

PCA—patient-controlled analgesia

PCO₂—partial pressure of carbon dioxide

PCP—*Pneumocystis jiroveci* pneumonia (formerly *Pneumocystis carinii* pneumonia), primary care physician

PD—peritoneal dialysis

PE—pulmonary embolism

PEEP—positive end-expiratory pressure

PERRLA—pupils equal, round, reactive to light and accommodation

PET—postural emission tomography

PFT—pulmonary function tests

pH—hydrogen ion concentration (level of acid/base)

PID—pelvic inflammatory disease

PKD—polycystic kidney disease

PKU—phenylketonuria

PMDD—premenstrual dysphoric disorder

PMS—premenstrual syndrome

PN—parenteral nutrition

PND—paroxysmal nocturnal dyspnea

PO, po—by mouth

PO₂—partial pressure of oxygen

PPD—positive purified protein derivative (of tuberculin)

PPN—partial parenteral nutrition

PRN, prn—as needed, whenever necessary

pro time—prothrombin time

PSA—prostate-specific antigen

psi—pounds per square inch

PSP—phenolsulfonphthalein

PT—physical therapy, prothrombin time

PTCA—percutaneous transluminal coronary angioplasty

PTH—parathyroid hormone

PTT—partial thromboplastin time

PUD—peptic ulcer disease

PVC—premature ventricular contraction

q—every

QA—quality assurance

qh—every hour

q 2 h—every 2 hours

q 4 h—every 4 hours

qid—four times a day

qs—quantity sufficient

R—rectal temperature, respirations, roentgen

RA—rheumatoid arthritis

RAI—radioactive iodine

RAIU—radioactive iodine uptake

RAS—reticular activating system

RBBB—right bundle branch block

RBC—red blood cell or count

RCA—right coronary artery

RDA—recommended dietary allowance

resp—respirations

RF—rheumatic fever, rheumatoid factor

Rh—antigen on blood cell indicated by + or –

RIND—reversible ischemic neurologic deficit

RLQ—right lower quadrant

RN—registered nurse

RNA—ribonucleic acid

R/O, r/o—rule out, to exclude

ROM—range of motion (of joint)

RUQ—right upper quadrant

Rx—prescription

s—without

S. or Sig.—(Signa) to write on label

SA—sinoatrial node

SaO$_2$—systemic arterial oxygen saturation (%)

sat sol—saturated solution

SBE—subacute bacterial endocarditis

SDA—same-day admission

SDS—same-day surgery

sed rate—sedimentation rate

SGOT—serum glutamic-oxaloacetic transaminase (*see* AST)

SGPT—serum glutamic-pyruvic transaminase (*see* ALT)

SI—International System of Units

SIADH—syndrome of inappropriate antidiuretic hormone

SIDS—sudden infant death syndrome

SL—sublingual

SLE—systemic lupus erythematosus

SOB—short of breath

sol—solution

SMBG—self-monitoring blood glucose

SMR—submucous resection

sp gr—specific gravity

spec.—specimen

SSKI—saturated solution of potassium iodide

stat—immediately

STI—sexually transmitted infection

subcut, subQ—subcutaneous

Sx—symptoms

Syr.—syrup

T—temperature, thoracic (to be followed by the number designating specific thoracic vertebra)

T&A—tonsillectomy and adenoidectomy

tabs—tablets

TB—tuberculosis

T&C—type and crossmatch

TED—thromboembolic device (compression stockings)

temp—temperature

TENS—transcutaneous electrical nerve stimulation

TIA—transient ischemic attack

TIBC—total iron binding capacity

tid—three times a day

tinct, tr.—tincture

TMJ—temporomandibular joint

tPA, TPA—tissue plasminogen activator

TPN—total parenteral nutrition

TPR—temperature, pulse, respiration

TQM—total quality management

TSE—testicular self-examination

TSH—thyroid-stimulating hormone

tsp—teaspoon

TSS—toxic shock syndrome

TURP—transurethral prostatectomy

UA—urinalysis

ung—ointment (unguent)

URI—upper respiratory tract infection

UTI—urinary tract infection

VAD—venous access device

VDRL—Venereal Disease Research Laboratory (test for syphilis)

VF, Vfib—ventricular fibrillation

VPC—ventricular premature complexes

VS, vs—vital signs

VSD—ventricular septal defect

VT—ventricular tachycardia

WBC—white blood cell, white blood count

WHO—World Health Organization

wt—weight

INDEX OF GENERIC MEDICATION NAMES

abacavir/lamivudine, 53

acetaminophen hydrocodone, 19

acetaminophen, 9

acyclovir, 55

adalimumab, 225

ADH (antidiuretic hormone), 295

albuterol sulfate, 255

alendronate, 187

allopurinol, 223

alprazolam, 215

alteplase, 31

aluminum hydroxide, 145

amikacin, 43

amiodarone HCl, 95

amitriptyline, 199

amlodipine, 117

amoxicillin, 43

amoxicillin/clavulanate, 45

amphetamine/dextroamphetamine, 211

amphotericin B, 47

ampicillin, 43

antidiuretic hormone (ADH), 295

antipyrine/benzocaine/glycerin otic solution, 249

apixaban, 25

aripiprazole, 209

aspirin, 11

atenolol, 111

atorvastatin calcium, 103

azithromycin, 67

baclofen, 231

beclomethasone, 5

benazepril HCl, 83

benzocaine/glycerin/antipyrine otic solution, 249

benzonatate, 253

benztropine, 235

bisoprolol, 113

brimonidine tartrate, 247

budesonide/formoterol, 257

bumetanide, 121

buprenorphine/naloxone, 15

bupropion HCl, 203

buspirone, 191

calcitonin salmon, 187

calcium carbonate, 145

captopril, 85

carbamazepine, 33

carbidopa/levodopa, 235

carbonyl iron, 265

carisoprodol, 231

carvedilol, 113

cefazolin, 59

cefdinir, 61

cefepime, 61

ceftriaxone, 61

cefuroxime, 59

celecoxib, 11
cephalexin, 59
cetirizine HCl, 1
chamomile (herbal), 177
chlordiazepoxide, 191
chlorthalidone, 125
cholecalciferol (aqueous
  vitamin D), 271
cimetidine, 157
ciprofloxacin, 63
cisplatin, 75
citalopram, 195
clarithromycin, 67
clavulanate/amoxicillin, 45
clindamycin, 65
clomiphene citrate, 303
clonazepam, 215
clonidine, 101
clopidogrel, 79
codeine, 17
colchicine, 223
conjugated estrogens, 301
co-trimoxazole (sulfamethoxaz-
  ole/trimethoprim), 69
cromolyn sodium, 261
cyanocobalamin, 273
cyclobenzaprine, 233
cyclophosphamide, 77

dabigatran, 27
darbepoetin alfa, 263
dexamethasone/tobramycin,
  247

dextroamphetamine/ampheta-
  mine, 211
diazepam, 217
diclofenac sodium, 227
digoxin, 121
diltiazem HCl, 117
diphenhydramine, 1
disulfiram, 261
divalproex sodium, 33
dobutamine, 291
donepezil, 237
dopamine, 293
dorzolamide HCl, 241
doxazosin mesylate, 87
doxepin, 201
doxycycline hyclate, 71
drospirenone/ethinyl estradiol,
  297
DTaP vaccine, 277
duloxetine HCl, 193

echinacea (herbal), 179
emtricitabine/tenofovir, 55
enalapril, 85
enoxaparin, 27
epinephrine, 293
epoetin alfa, 263
ergocalciferol, 273
erythromycin, 69
escitalopram oxalate, 195
esomeprazole, 163
estradiol (oral), 301
estradiol valerate, 301

estrogens, conjugated, 301
etanercept, 227
ethinyl estradiol/drospirenone, 297
ethinyl estradiol/ethynodiol, 297
ethinyl estradiol/norethindrone, 299
ethynodiol/ethinyl estradiol, 297
exenatide, 133
ezetimibe, 103

famotidine, 159
fenofibrate, 105
fentanyl, 17
ferric gluconate complex, 267
ferrous sulfate, 267
feverfew (herbal), 179
fexofenadine, 3
finasteride, 175
flecainide, 95
flu vaccine, 281
fluconazole, 47
fluocinonide, 131
fluoxetine HCl, 197
fluticasone, 7
folic acid, 275
formoterol/budesonide, 257
furosemide, 123

gabapentin, 35
galantamine, 239

garlic (herbal), 181
gemfibrozil, 105
gentamicin, 43
ginger (herbal), 181
gingko (herbal), 183
ginseng (herbal), 183
glimepiride, 133
glipizide, 135
glucagon, 143
glyburide, 135
glycerin, 159
glycerin/antipyrine/benzocaine otic solution, 249
guaifenesin, 259

Haemophilus influenzae type B (HIB) vaccine, 277
haloperidol, 205
heparin, 29
hepatitis A vaccine, 279
hepatitis B vaccine, 279
HIB (Haemophilus influenzae type B) vaccine, 277
HPV vaccine, 281
human papillomavirus (HPV) vaccine, 281
hydralazine HCl, 101
hydrochlorothiazide, 127
hydrocodone/acetaminophen, 19
hydrocortisone, 71
hydrocortisone/neomycin/polymyxin otic, 249

hydromorphone, 19
hydroxocobalamin, 275
hydroxychloroquine, 49
hydroxyzine, 3
hyoscyamine, 147

ibuprofen, 13
indomethacin, 229
influenza vaccine, 277
influenza vaccine, 281
insulin aspart, 139
insulin glargine, 141
insulin lispro, 139
insulin, regular, 143
insulin-isophane suspension (NPH insulin), 141
ipratropium, 255
isoniazid, 51
isosorbide dinitrate, 93

ketoconazole, 129

lactulose, 161
lamivudine/abacavir, 53
lamotrigine, 35
lansoprazole, 165
latanoprost, 243
levobunolol, 245
levodopa/carbidopa, 235
levofloxacin, 63
levothyroxine (T4), 189
lidocaine HCl, 97
lisdexamfetamine dimesylate, 213

lisinopril, 87
lithium, 219
loperamide HCl, 147
loratadine, 5
lorazepam, 217
losartan, 91
lovastatin, 107

magnesium sulfate, 37
measles, mumps, & rubella (MMR) vaccine, 283
meclizine, 149
medroxyprogesterone acetate, 303
meloxicam, 13
memantine HCl, 239
meningococcal vaccine, 283
metformin HCl, 137
methadone, 21
methocarbamol, 233
methotrexate, 77
methylphenidate HCl, 213
methylprednisolone, 73
metoclopramide HCl, 149
metolazone, 127
metoprolol, 115
metronidazole, 51
minoxidil (topical), 265
mirabegron, 171
mirtazapine, 203
misoprostol, 153

MMR vaccine, 283

mometasone, 7

montelukast, 251

morphine, 21

naloxone HCl, 269

naloxone/buprenorphine, 15

naltrexone, 271

naproxen, 15

neomycin/polymyxin/
    hydrocortisone otic, 249

niacin (nicotinic acid), 107

nicardipine, 289

nicotinic acid (niacin), 107

nifedipine, 119

nitrofurantoin, 177

nitroglycerin, 93

nitroprusside, 291

norepinephrine, 295

norethindrone, 299

norethindrone/ethinyl estradiol,
    299

nortriptyline, 201

NPH insulin (insulin-isophane
    suspension), 141

nystatin, 129

olanzapine, 211

omeprazole, 165

ondansetron, 151

oseltamivir, 57

oxybutynin chloride, 169

oxycodone, 23

pancrelipase, 163

pantoprazole, 167

paroxetine HCl, 197

PCV13 vaccine, 285

penicillin, 43

phenobarbital, 37

phentermine, 157

phenytoin, 39

pioglitazone HCl, 137

piperacillin/tazobactam, 45

piroxicam, 229

pneumococcal conjugate
    (PCV13) vaccine, 285

pneumococcal polysaccharide
    vaccine (PPSV23), 285

polio vaccine, 287

polyethylene glycol, 161

polymyxin/hydrocortisone/
    neomycin otic, 249

potassium chloride, 269

PPSV23 vaccine, 285

prasugrel, 81

pravastatin, 109

prazosin HCl, 89

prednisolone, 73

prednisone, 75

pregabalin, 39

probenecid, 225

procainamide, 97

promethazine, 151

propofol, 25

propranolol HCl, 115

K

quetiapine, 207
quinidine, 99
quinine sulfate, 49

rabeprazole, 167
regular insulin, 143
rifampin, 53
risedronate, 189
risperidone, 207
rivaroxaban, 29
rivastigmine, 239
rosuvastatin calcium, 109
rotavirus vaccine, 287

salmeterol, 257
selegiline, 237
sertraline, 199
sildenafil citrate, 173
simethicone, 153
simvastatin, 111
sitagliptin, 139
sotalol, 99
spironolactone, 125
St. John's wort (herbal), 185
sucralfate, 155
sulfamethoxazole/trimethoprim
   (co-trimoxazole), 69
sulfasalazine, 155
sumatriptan, 41

T4 (levothyroxine), 189
tadalafil, 173
tamoxifen, 79

tamsulosin HCl, 169
tazobactam/piperacillin, 45
Td vaccine, 277
Tdap vaccine, 277
temazepam, 219
tenofovir/emtricitabine, 55
terazosin HCl, 89
terbutaline sulfate, 259
theophylline, 251
ticagrelor, 81
ticlopidine HCl, 83
timolol, 245
tiotropium, 253
tobramycin, 43
tobramycin/dexamethasone,
   247
tolterodine tartrate, 171
topiramate, 41
torsemide, 123
tramadol, 23
travoprost, 243
trazodone, 205
triamcinolone acetonide, 131
triamcinolone, 9
trimethoprim/sulfamethoxazole
   (co-trimoxazole), 69

valacyclovir HCl, 57
valerian (herbal), 185
valproate, 33
valproic acid, 33
valsartan, 91
vancomycin, 65

vardenafil, 175

varicella vaccine, 289

vasopressin (antidiuretic
  hormone), 295

venlafaxine, 193

verapamil HCl, 119

warfarin, 31

zaleplon, 221

ziprasidone HCl, 209

zolmitriptan, 241

zolpidem tartrate, 221

K